# USMLE SMASHER

## A Smart Guide to
## Smash USMLE Clinical Skills

## K.G. Paul MD

**To order additional copies of this book, contact:**
Xlibris Corporation
1-888-795-4274
www.Xlibris.com
Orders@Xlibris.com
49888

# USMLE SMASHER

# CONTENTS

# SmartDoc

medical books

New York London Delhi Shanghai

Our Father's God! To Thee,
Author Of Liberty,
To Thee We Sing;
Long May Our Land Be Bright
With Freedom's Holy Light;
Protect Us By Thy Might,
Great God, Our King!


Dedicated to my wife Dr. Nini Thomas and all other physicians,residents,
and future residents serving the people of the United States of America

# 1

# Introducing USMLE SMASHER

In common usage, a SMASHER has many meanings. But two particular definitions caught my attention before I chose it as the title of this book. In physical sciences, the atomic smasher has two functions. First it increases the kinetic energy of the charged particles.As I write these words, scientists at CERN, the European Organization for Nuclear Research, are building Large Hadron Collider. LHC will be the world's largest atomic smasher as it uses an unprecedented peak energy of 14 trillion electron volts to smash two beams of protons together, and in the process, to discover new types of smaller particles, known as quarks.

When I heard about Large Hadron Collider, I was bemused by the importance of understanding the microstructures of the atom in order to decipher the macrostructure of our universe. I think similar principle holds importance even in the health care: it starts with laying the foundation with basic principles of physician-patient communication and then building the edifice of patient care on the top of it. That is where this book starts. Patient Encounters are intended to make all the bricks of patient communication available to the physician to work upon.

Second, that atomic smasher breaks the atom into small pieces. This book is written with the same purpose in mind. It dissects the USMLE Clinical Skills Examination into small components and explain the basic principles to score high in each component.

My second definition of Smasher comes from the world of sports. In sports, to smash means to hit a ball in a forceful stroke. I think the first principle to achieve success is to unleash your best shot at the target with all the force you can muster in the given time. Perhaps the greatest baseball player in history, Babe Ruth once described how he hit home runs, "How to hit home runs: I swing as hard as I can . . . . I swing big, with everything I've got. I hit big or I miss big. I like to live as big as I can"

I hope this book will help you deliver your best shot at USMLE Clinical Skills, to smash it and then to realize your dreams in medical profession.

Please send me your comments, corrections and criticisms to *drkgpaul@gmail.com*

I wish you all the best,
K.G.Paul MD

# 2

# Check List

I have filled the application form on the website: NBME or ECFMG ☐
I have a government-issued photo identification to present at the test center for
   identification (If you do not have one, start now to get one, it takes time) ☐
I have a white lab coat and a stethoscope ☐
I have received the notification of registration ☐
I have scheduled my test date ☐
I have prepared a study plan for this test ☐
I have learned the history taking techniques ☐
I have mastered all basic physical examination methods ☐
I know how to counsel patients for common clinical problems ☐
I have practised doing my patient encounters within time limit ☐
I have memorized the important mnemonics ☐
I am aware of the test procedure, regulations and requirements ☐
I have planned my travel to the test center ☐
I have reserved my flight ticket, bus ticket or train ticket (whatever necessary) ☐
I have reserved my room in the nearby hotel (if necessary) ☐

Before leaving home:

I have packed my admission permit and government issued photo identification ☐
I have packed my white lab coat and stethoscope before leaving for the test center ☐

# 3

## Things To Remember

### DOs

☺ Read the doorway information carefully along with the specific instructions regarding the tasks you are supposed to perform

☺ Knock on the door before you enter the examination room

☺ Introduce yourself to the patient

☺ Always look into the patient's eyes when you speak to them

☺ Always start your patient interview with open-ended questions

☺ Use simple, clear words in framing your questions

☺ Use transitional questions while moving from one topic to the other

☺ Always drape the patient before starting your physical examination

☺ Always wash your hands before examining the patient

☺ Always answer the patient's questions, if you do not know the answer, say, 'I don't know'.

☺ In your physical examination, explain to the patient what you are going to do before doing it

☺ After your physical examination, help the patient put their gown back on

☺ Explain your findings and tentative diagnosis to the patient

☺ Explain to the patient about the investigations and laboratory tests you are going to order

☺ Give a brief conclusion/counseling at the end of your patient encounter

☺ Ask the patient whether they have any questions for you

☺ Thank the patient for their cooperation, once you finish the encounter and about to leave

☺ Do a fundus examination in all diabetic patients

☺ Carefully look for the abnormal signs in your physical examination

☺ Remember to examine the abdomen in the correct order: inspection, auscultation, percussion, and palpation

☺ Be a good listener and pay attention to the patient while they are talking with you

☺ Do complement the patient if it is sincere

# DON'Ts

- ☹ Do not try to cram new material on the day of or the day before the test.
- ☹ Do not use medical terminology in your conversation with the patient
- ☹ Do not examine the patient through the gown
- ☹ Do not rush or compel the patient
- ☹ Do not give false reassurance about the outcome of the disease
- ☹ Do not perform a pelvic, genital, rectal, female breast and corneal reflex tests
- ☹ Do not get perplexed even if you feel you have 'messed up' two or three cases
- ☹ Do not talk too fast that your patient cannot understand you
- ☹ Do not jabber
- ☹ Do not talk down
- ☹ Do not make fun of the patient's questions, answers, behavior etc.
- ☹ Do not contradict the patient
- ☹ Do not ask embarrassing personal questions
- ☹ Do not make tactless comments
- ☹ Do not use "Mr" before your name in your introduction to the patient
- ☹ Do not repeat painful maneuvers.
- ☹ Do not give the patient more information than they can handle
- ☹ Do not reenter the examination room, once you go outside, to ask 'forgotten' questions in history or to perform 'missed' tests in physical examination. Before you leave the patient examination room make sure that you have finished everything relevant to that case
- ☹ Do not waste your time with rechecking the vital signs given on the doorway information sheet, unless you are specifically asked to do so.
- ☹ Do not perform a 'head to toe' pattern of physical examination. You should be able to do a focused physical examination with in 5 to 6 minutes.
- ☹ Do not mark on the patient's body during your physical examination.
- ☹ Do not make twitchy mannerisms—pulling at your hair, pursing your mouth, wrinkling your brow etc.
- ☹ Do not interrupt the patient while they are doing the talking
- ☹ Do not show your nervousness or anxiety in front of the patient
- ☹ Do not look at the big clock on the wall in the examination room, repeatedly.
- ☹ Do not hesitate to say such gracious words like 'please' and 'thank you' to the SP
- ☹ Do not link positive remark with a negative one (e.g. You are taking good care of your diabetes, but you neglected.)
- ☹ Do not ask multiple choice questions, ask one question at a time
- ☹ Do not ask leading questions
- ☹ Do not close your open-ended questions with another closed-ended question (e.g. Tell me about your pain? Is it severe?)
- ☹ Do not leave the examination room without saying goodbye to the patient
- ☹ Do not linger at the door after your conclusion

☹ Do not show off your medical knowledge to the SP using medical knowledge. Translate your medical vocabulary into lay terminology before conveying to the patient

☹ Do not keep your hands on patient's head while doing the ophthalmoscopic examination.

☹ Do not write less familiar abbreviations in your patient note.

☹ Do not write treatment plans, referrals, and management plans in your diagnostic work up

# 4

## Success Tips

An old Chinese proverb says, *"Tell me, I'll forget. Show me, I may remember. But involve me, I'll understand and master.* USMLE Step-2 Clinical Skills is a unique test with its own characteristics and keeping them in your perspective while preparing for this examination is the key to success. This chapter focuses on the main components of an effective preparation to succeed in this test. Synchronizing various parts of your preparation according to a few time-tested guide lines help you habituate yourself to perform and pass this test with an imperturbable demeanor. Try to apply the following principles to your preparation.

1.  **Practice! Practice! Practice!**

    Remember that USMLE Clinical Skills Examination is not as easy as it would seem. Your absolute key to success in this test is practicing with patients in a real clinical setting or, at least, with someone who can portray as your standardized patient. *All your study material tell you what to ask in history, what to look for in physical examination and where to look, but they can never replace practice.* Find a study partner or friend, who can portray patients in a realistic way and every day, practice at least one case with them: history taking and physical examination, always being aware of time limit. However, the best preparation is to see the actual patients in a real clinical setting such as a medical clinic or hospital, under the supervision of a competent physician, who can critique your performance.

    Since USMLE Step-2 CS is designed to simulate an actual clinical experience, the more clinical experience and practice you have, the more comfortable you will feel during the patient encounter in this test. If you do not have a helpmate around you, try for a phone study partner. Following a fixed time frame, discuss the cases everyday over the phone, while you are acting as the physician and your conversant acting as the standardized patient. Studying with another person or with a small group, enhances your learning a lot. But do not join a group, which rises your anxiety level or is not serious about Step-2 CS. For instance, do not take a student preparing for USMLE Step-3 or Step-1 or

Step-2 CK as your study partner. USMLE Step-2 CS is a lot different examination from other USMLE examinations. Again, what you need is practice, especially if you are out of touch with the patients recently.

2.  **Develop a study plan and stick to it**

    Allow plenty of time for the study and revision of important material. Many students preparing for this test are bewildered with a question, *How many days do I need to study for this test?* Though this is a subjective decision, for a medical student or graduate, who is adequately trained in his or her medical school, approximately thirty days are sufficient for a confident preparation for this test. However, this decision must be made carefully by the student himself/herself individually lest they endanger their preparation and outcome of this test.

    Stick to your study plan with a steady pace. Plan what you will need to study and when and over how many days you are trying to learn the required tasks. Do not rush, but study chapter after chapter, form the fundamental clinical knowledge base, develop the basic clinical skills and review the common diseases, their symptoms and signs, and the relevant physical examination. While it is important to learn the topics essential to pass this examination, one tends to forget the most vital points as the days of preparation progresses toward the day of examination. That is why you need a strategy to remember what you've learned. It is also extremely important to analyze how your daily study is relevant to your examination and to maintain the coherence between the topics of study and the things tested in the examination

3.  **Organize your material for a parallel study.**

    Allot the greatest amount of your time to the most important topics of the test. Rather than studying history taking, physical examination, and patient note writing sequentially, follow a parallel study plan. For instance, study the history taking of a particular system in the morning, the physical examination of that system in the afternoon, and then it's patient note writing in the evening. This mode of study help you concrete your thinking in the mode of the actual examination.

4.  **Take breaks**

    Anxiety is your most ruthless enemy in this test. It is usual that you experience some level of nervousness before this test because of the cost of failure in terms of the fee, impact on the residency interviews, and loss of time, sometimes, a full resident year. But, remember nervousness actually devastates your preparation and minimizes your chances of success. Therefore, do not allow your anxiety to run the show. Take charge of the preparation with an attitude of self-confidence. Take breaks for relaxation. Taking deep breaths, remembering your past academic victories, rotating your shoulders are some of the well known techniques to relax yourself and boost your confidence level.

5. **Face the test with confidence**

   As mentioned earlier, anxiety and nervousness destroy everything you planned for. Anxiety is like a double-edged sword. A little anxiety is a good thing. Some level of anxiety, which is usual for all of us, can be channeled into a motivating force that help us energize, focus, and prepare well, but too much of tension will paralyze and incapacitate us, for the bad results. Therefore, it is important to face this test with confidence. After all, you have been exposed to the components of this examination—history taking, physical examination and patient note writing—ever since you entered into the medical school. Beside you have finished the United States Medical Licensing Examination Step-1 in order to get the eligibility to sit for this test. Taking your medical school experience and the Step-1 success into the context, with good preparation, passing Step-2 Clinical Skills should not be a difficult task to overcome. *The pass in Step-1 is an attestation that you have enough cognitive skills to appear for this examination.* However, on the other hand, it is equally important to recognize the fact that your score in Step-1 is not a card of assurance that you are going to pass this test. To say that using an example, a student with 96 percentile score in Step-1 might fail in clinical skills examination due to lack of preparation and practice, which, sometimes, is bred by over-confidence generated from a high score in Steps. Succinctly, it is your practice and preparation for this test—not your scores in other Steps—which determine your success. Completion of USMLE Step-2 Clinical Knowledge in not required to perform well in Step-2 Clinical Skills either. Above all, avoid thinking of yourself in a negative sense.

6. **Learn the mnemonics**

   Completing history taking, physical examination and counseling the patient within 15 minutes is an awesome task. Time flies away very quickly during patient encounters. To barrage yourself against the tides of anxiety related to the tasks, learn the essential mnemonics given in this book. They enhance your memory and speed of performance in the real test.

7. **Improve your English proficiency**

   One of the components of this test is proficiency in English language, which will be assessed by the standardized patients. Excellence in clinical skills does not compensate a poor English language proficiency. It is also important to recognize that having English as mother language or the language of one's upbringing is not a guarantee that he or she has English proficiency. For example, even an American-born student may fail to communicate his or her ideas effectively to the patient while a student from a non-English background may have troubles with pronunciations. Thus, regardless of one's upbringing, it is important to improve their English language skills: Transforming thoughts into meaningful sentences using accurate grammar, identifying words that clearly communicate one's point of view, feelings and ideas, learning to pronounce those words clearly and confidently, spelling the words correctly and writing legibly if you are planning to write your patient note rather typing on the computer. If you are uncertain of your English language proficiency, consider taking TOEFL or/and TSE (Test of Spoken English) as screening tests prior to applying for the USMLE Step 2 CS.

8.  **Revise your previously studied material as frequently as possible**
    It is important to recognize the truth that human beings forget 46% of what they read after one day, 79% after 14 days, and 81% after 28 days. Thus, if you start your one-month study plan today, you will have forgotten 81% of what you have studied today by the end of your study plan. Thus, it is essential to review your previous study regularly to get the maximum benefits from your study plan.

9.  **Familiarize with the test procedure**
    Lastly, familiarization with the test procedures is as essential as the studying for the test. Many students fail because of their non-acquaintance with the testing procedures and regulations. Please read the orientation material often and watch the videos in the CD to get familiarized with the testing procedure. Synchronize your preparation with hoarding essential information about the testing procedures and regulations.

10. **Make preparations in advance**
    Finally make preparations for your test well in advance, at least 6 months on hand, because there is an year-round demand for test dates, test centers, flight tickets, hotel rooms, car rentals etc

## THE DAY BEFORE THE TEST

1.  **Relax yourself!** : On the day before the test, you must relax yourself from all anxiety. Avoid cramming new material at this time. Trying to learn new techniques, maneuvers, formulas, mnemonics on the day before the test can easily produce anxiety.
2.  If you are traveling a long distance, consider **arriving** in the test-town **at least a day before the test.** For example, do not plan to take a morning flight to Philadelphia on the day of the test. Also, do not plan to arrive at the test center through a long-hour driving, which might exhaust you. Amtrak, Greyhound and some airlines are becoming synonymous with delay and disruptions. Therefore, do not plan to travel on the day of the test. Get the information about restaurants, motels, and weather conditions of the city of your test center.

3. **Review major concepts** of history taking, physical examination and doctor-patient communication. This should be limited to the material you have already studied during your preparation. Again, attempting to crash learn new material at this pivotal time may interfere with your recall of material you have already mastered.

4. If you completed your study plan, **do something relaxing** that refreshes your mind. This does not affect your performance in the test.

5. **Avoid calling** any friends you know to be **'tension creators'**. They might ask you whether you have learned 'glabellar reflex' in case if you get an elderly patient tomorrow as a case under neurological diseases or 'Do you know how to explain Weil-Felix reaction if your patient ask about it tomorrow?' These unnecessary questions actually elevate your anxiety.

6. On the day before the test **do not eat** foods that are traditionally known to produce 'loose stools', for example milk shakes, fruit salads, spicy foods or any other foods that you have identified in your personal experience to be **bowel stimulators**. They may wreak havoc during the test time as you get constant urge to run to the restroom.

7. **Get plenty of sleep** the night before the test—the better rested you are, the more likely you will be able to perform at your best. Also, do not plan any travel or driving that rob you of a sound sleep on the night before the test.

# THE DAY OF THE TEST

**Before the Test:**

1. **Get up early** from the bed.
2. Try to **engage in a relaxation activity** the hour before the exam.
3. Have **moderate breakfast** and avoid excessive amounts of coffee, which is known to cause light-headedness and jitteriness on the day of the test.
4. **Avoid cramming new material**, which will cloud the concepts, which you have already learned.
5. You might need a shower, but **wear comfortable, professional clothing** and a white laboratory or clinic coat. Carry your stethoscope with you. All other necessary medical equipment is provided in the examination rooms.
6. Take your **admission permit** and government-issued **photo identification** with you, before you leave your motel or home.
7. **Plan to arrive** at the test center no more than thirty minutes prior to your scheduled test. Take **traffic** in that area into your travel plan. Get correct driving directions from your home to the test center.
8. After arriving at the test center, please **follow the instructions of the test center staff** at all times. Many a time they give you essential directions, you should not miss.

9. **Sign the confidentiality agreement at the test center**, which stipulates that you will not reveal the patient information to anyone over the phone or internet chat room or discussion forum, or in any other form at any time.

10. **Carry only necessary personal items** with you to the center, where you can store them in a small, open storage cubicle, assigned to you. Do not carry other luggage with you, which can not be stored in the test center.

11. **Avoid contacting** your friends, who are known as **'anxiety generators'**, lest they might ask you, 'How do you counsel the patient with Canavan's disease?'

12. If your waiting for the test causes anxiety, **distract yourself** by reading a newspaper or Step-2 Orientation manual.

13. After arriving at the test center, **make sure** that your **admission permit** and **photo identification** are in your pocket or purse.

14. **Do not take your friends, family or spouses to the test center** because there will be no waiting facilities for them.

15. The test begins with an on-site orientation. **Concentrate on the orientation** to get familiarized with the examination procedures, regulations and equipment in each examination room. This is your last opportunity to get familiarized to the medical equipment you may need inside the examination room. So, practice with that equipment thoroughly before going into the examination room.

16. Consider making one final **visit to the rest room** before starting the test encounters!

## AFTER YOU START THE TEST

1. **Time just flies away** once you start your first patient encounter.

2. **Do not write** anything on the scrap paper **until the announcement to do so**

3. **Carefully read the information** on the doorway information sheet.

4. Beside information about the patient's name, his age, his chief complaint and vital signs, there will be specific instruction on what you are supposed to do inside the examination room. **This information varies from case to case**. Do not neglect to read this essential information written on the doorway information sheet.

5. **Do not chew gum** while the test is going on. It will affect the clarity of your questions during your history taking. Also, for the general public, speaking to someone while chewing gum is a sign of carelessness.

6. Before you enter into the examination room, write down the essential information about the patient and **your mnemonic** on your scrap paper. This scrap or blank paper will be provided by the test center proctors.

7. **Knock the door** before you enter the examination room.

8. Perform your patient encounter **decently and professionally**.

9. Do not put too much emphasis on completed cases. Without argument, every student will forget doing a few essential things in some of their cases. **Try not**

**to repeat the same mistakes in subsequent cases.** For example, if you forgot to ask the duration of illness in one case, try to remember to ask about it in the next case. But, while facing one patient encounter, never think about the questions you forgot to ask in the previous patient encounter. Such a recollection will rob you of your thinking, which is essential to frame your questions for the current patient encounter. **Always concentrate on the case on which you are working**.

10. **Enjoy your breaks** for relaxation, refreshments and restrooms.

11. **Do not drink fluids too much,** which may force you for frequent restroom visits.

12. During the breaks **do not discuss the cases** with your fellow candidates. Based on the patient encounters you've finished, do not announce your 'pass' or 'fail' result to other examinees, either.

13. Enjoy the refreshments during the breaks. **Do not ponder on the mistakes** you have done in the completed cases.

14. If you encounter any problem, do not waste your time worrying about what to do. Notify the test center staff of any problems. Do not hesitate to **call the proctor** if you develop any problem at any part of your testing session. Just raise your hand or call them.

# AFTER THE TEST

1. **Recollect your belongings** from your storage cubicle in the test center.

2. **Enjoy the reward you promised yourself** after test—whether you did the test well or not.

3. Remember **Success is never ending** and **failure is never final**

# 5

# Patient Encounters

This chapter consists of 11 Patient Encounters, which represent the wide variety of cases encountered in Step-2 CS examination. The readers are not expected to follow the exact pattern used by the physician interviewing the patients in these cases. These cases are only intended to reflect the most common flow of patient encounter in the Step-2 CS examination.

1. Abdominal pain
2. Urinary incontinence
3. Chest pain
4. Weight gain (depression)
5. Diarrhea
6. Diabetes medication refill
7. SCUBA diving complete medical form
8. Pediatric diarrhea
9. Vaginal discharge
10. Headache
11. Telephone Interview

# FIRST PATIENT ENCOUNTER

**Mrs. Jacqueline Kemp, a 34-year old female complaining of severe abdominal pain**
**Blood pressure = 110/70 Heart Rate = 94 Respirations = 18 Temperature = 98.7**

**Perform a focused history and physical examination on this patient. After leaving the room, complete your patient note on the form provided.**

| | |
|---|---|
| *Dr: Hello, good morning, I am Dr. Paul. Are you, Mrs.Kemp?*<br>Pt: Yes, I am glad to know you<br>*Dr: Thank you, I'm glad to know you too.* | Start your encounter with a **KISS**<br>**K—Knock on the door**<br>(Knocking on the door is the first display of your respect towards the patient)<br>**I—Introduce yourself and Identify the patient**<br>(introduce yourself in a clear voice, do not mumble, do not mispronounce patient's name, if you can't pronounce well, ask patient's help to verify. Use patient's last name. Since you are not the patient's friend, it would demonstrate lack of respect to use his or her first name during an initial interview.<br>**S—Smile,**<br>(smiling is the first step to endear yourself to any stranger)<br>**S—Shake hand and Sit near**<br>(Shake hand is the first physical contact you make with the patient; Sit at the patient's level in a position where you can be easily seen and heard.) |
| *Dr: Mrs. Kemp, let us have a small chat regarding your problem. I would like to put this cloth on you so that you feel can more comfortable. Is that all right with you?*<br>Pt: No problem, doctor | After KISS, do RED<br>**R—Relax**<br>Do not get hasty which makes the patient uneasy to interact with you. Your clinic is not the natural habitiat of the patient. He or she is already in the stress of illness, meeting a new doctor, unknown outcomes. If the physician is not relaxed, that only produces a barrier between the physician and the patient. |

**E—Eye contact**

Eye contact with the patient is the first step in your non-verbal communication. However, good eye contact does not mean staring fixedly at the patient, which only make the individual feel uncomfortable.

**D—Drape**, it is one way to make patient more comfortable. Inquire about and arrange for the patient's comfort before getting started and continue to consider his or her comfort during the course of your history and physical examination Remember actual physical examination starts right from the moment you walked into the room. You can start observing patient's posture, affect, skin color, hygiene, behavior and mental status.

*Mr. Kemp, I would like to talk to you today in order to get some information about why you're here and then to examine you. Will that be all right?*
Yes, first of all, I'm here mainly because of pain in my lower tummy. I am afraid I am going to die.
*(doctor nods his head),I understand your concerns, Mrs. Kemp,Is your pain one sided or both sided?*
It is on my right side.

Physician told what he is going to do and also obtained patient's consent for that. He demonstrated interest in and respect for the person. Do not say, *'I was told to take history and do a physical'* or *'This examination requires me to do a history taking and a physical. So, let us start'* or *'I was sent to take your history and do a physical'.* These statements reflect that you are not really interested in the patient.
Start your conversation with CPR
CPR—Chief complaint
Chief complaint is the main reason the patient came for medical help. Record it verbatim in the patient's own words.
**Common questions to elicit chief complaints:**
*What brought you to the hospital?*
*How can I help you today?*
*Can you tell me about your problem?*
*Please tell me about the main problem you feel is wrong*

*Let us start with discussing your main problem today. What problem brought you today?*

*I'm glad you came in today. What bothers you today?*

You can respond to the patient in a way to indicate you have heard what he or she has said.

*How exactly did the pain start?*

Pt:Doctor, it started this morning around 8'o clock. I was preparing the lunch pack for my husband. I was walking to the refrigerator from our kitchen. Suddenly, I had a devastating pain in my lower tummy. I almost fainted when I landed into the arms of my husband. He brought me to the hospital immediately.

*Have you ever had anything like this before?*

No, doctor, never.

(Patient takes a pause and says)

I am frightened with this pain.

Dr: *I can see you are. Now, How is the progression of pain? Is it getting better, worse, or staying the same?*

This damn pain, sometimes increasing and sometimes decreasing.

*Do you have any other complaints beside pain in the abdomen?*

I also have bleeding through vagina

*How many pads were soaked?*

6

CPR—Present illness, History of

History of present illness is the evolution of patient's symptoms from the time the patient last fell 'well' until the present. Start with open-ended questions.

**Common questions to elaborate present illness:**

*Tell me more about your pain*

*Tell me how your headaches bother you*

*Can you tell me more about your chest pain?*

Do not interrupt the patient when they are talking. Verbal interruptions are the prominent manifestations of your inattentiveness and the lack of patience.

Duration of the problem helps you to decide whether the presenting condition is acute or chronic.

Using a pleasant voice, speak with clarity to communicate understandably.

Avoid vulgar, nonstandard or obsolete words in your conversation.

*I can see you are:* Acknowledge patient's feelings. Do not minimize them with responses like, 'it is just in your head' or 'you need to take your mind off it' or 'I'm sure it wasn't that bad'

*Did the bleeding start after the pain or before the pain?*
The bleeding started a few minutes after the abdominal pain.

*How is the progression of bleeding?*
it has been increasing

*What color best describes the bleeding you had?*
The bleeding is slight, dark and watery, looking like 'prune juice', I never had such a bleeding before, doctor.

*Are you sexually active?*
Pt: Yes

*Could you be pregnant?*
I don't know.

*When was your last menstrual period?*
Two months ago

*Did you undergo any medical tests to detect pregnancy?*
No, doctor.

Do not try to read your mentally framed, premature diagnosis into the patient's history. Open-ended questions provide a barrier to this temptation.

Suspect intraperitoneal bleeding due to rupture of ectopic pregnancy in an young lady presenting with amenorrhea, abdominal pain and vaginal bleeding

Ask about the number of pads soaked to estimate the amount of bleeding.
Try to find the association between different presenting symptoms of the patient

Determine the course of the illness

'Prune juice' bleeding should alert you to the possibility of ectopic pregnancy. Use closed-ended questions to obtain specific information from the patient. Closed-ended questions usually end with specific information from the patient, e.g. 'yes' or 'no'.

Think about pregnancy in every female patient of child bearing age

Ask about LMP in every female patient of child-bearing age

|  | In ectopic pregnancy, pregnancy test may be positive but not always |
|---|---|
| -*Can you think of any other symptoms that you've had lately?*<br>Woo (patient mumbles)<br>*How is your vision?*<br>Slightly blurry | **CPR** Review of Systems<br>A complete system-by-system ROS is not possible in CS-2 exam due to limited amount of time. Therefore, asking pertinent positives and pertinent negatives is more important than asking questions related to every system in the body. For example, asking for the presence of shortness of breath is more important in a patient with cough than enquiring about numbness in the feet<br>Woo: When patient does not know how to answer your general questions, frame your questions in more direct manner |
| *Are you feeling light-headed or faint?*<br>Yes, doctor<br><br>*Do you have pain in any other areas of your body?*<br>My right shoulder is also aching since this morning. | Suspect internal bleeding in a patient, who complains light-headedness in the presence of symptoms suggestive of ectopic pregnancy.<br><br>Shoulder pain may be due to internal bleeding, which irritates the diaphragm when the patient breathes in and out. |
| *Now, I would like to ask you a series of questions to understand your pain more clearly. Please show me exactly where it is hurting you?*<br>Here (The patient pointed her finger to the lower abdomen) | Use a transitional before you jump from one topic to the other.<br>For all pain complaints ask the mnemonic<br>LIQOR FAAA TRIFT;<br>L for Location |
| *On a scale of 1 to 10, if 1 is the least painful and 10 is the most painful what number would you assign for your pain?*<br>Probably 9 | LIQOR FAAA TRIFT<br>I for Intensity |

| | |
|---|---|
| *How would you describe your pain?* I can't find words, but it is getting the hell out of me. | LIQOR FAAA TRIFT Q for Quality |
| *How did your pain start, suddenly or slowly?* It started very suddenly as if something was blown up in my belly, doctor, I was afraid I was going to die | LIQOR FAAA TRIFT O for Onset Differential Diagnosis: Suspect the following when a young lady presents with sudden pain in her abdomen: 1. ectopic pregnancy 2. acute appendicitis 3. acute pelvic inflammatory disease 4. ruptured corpus luteum cyst 5. ruptured ovarian follicle 6. urinary calculi 7. aborting uterine pregnancy 8. aborting hydatiform mole |
| *Does the pain move to any other part of your body?* No | LIQOR FAAA TRIFT R for Radiation Do not use words like 'radiate', 'transmission'. Use simple words, which the patient can understand. Clues from the radiation of pain: 1. Ectopic pregnancy: pain does NOT radiate. 2. Pancreatitis: Deep epigastric pain with radiatiation to the back 3. Appendicitis: pain radiate from umbilical region to right lower quadrant 4. Aortic dissection: severe, persistent chest pain with radiation to the back. |
| *Does the pain stay all the time or does it come and go?* It is coming and going. | LIQOR FAAA TRIFT : F for Frequency Pain is intermittent in ectopic pregnancy |
| *Does anything make your pain worse?* it is more painful when I am walking | LIQOR FAAA TRIFT: A for Aggravating factors |

| | |
|---|---|
| *Does anything make your pain better?*<br>no doctor | LIQOR FAAA TRIFT: A for Alleviating factors |
| *Do you have any other symptoms beside abdominal pain and vaginal bleeding?*<br>I have backache for the last six hours. In fact, I wish I could sleep in the home rather visiting your office. | LIQOR FAAA TRIFT: A for Associated factors<br>Backache and sweating are common presentations in attacks of ectopic pregnancy |
| *So you got a very painful belly since this morning, right?*<br>Yes, doctor.<br>*Now, I need to ask you some more questions, OK, Have you had any injuries or accidents involving your belly?*<br>No, doctor | Verification: Use verifications to clarify the information with the patient.<br><br>LIQOR FAAA TRIFT: T for Trauma<br>Abdominal pain due to trauma in a young lady, should prompt you to think about the possibility of spousal abuse. |
| *Have you developed any rash, I mean any eruptions of spots on the skin recently?*<br>No | LIQOR FAAA TRIFT: R for Rash<br>Use vocabulary adapted to the level of the patient. If you speak out any difficult words, try to explain them to the patient immediately lest the patient get confused.<br>Suspect SLE in patients presenting with facial rash, fatigue and abdominal pain |
| *Have you been running a fever?*<br>No | LIQOR FAAA TRIFT: F for Fever<br>Fever might present in conditions like ectopic pregnancy |
| *Have you traveled anywhere recently?*<br>*No*<br><br>*Now, Mrs. Kemp, I would like to ask you about your health in general. Is it O.K with you?*<br>yes, doctor | LIQOR FAAA TRIFT: T for Travel<br>Foreign travel increases the risk of intestinal infection that may present with abdominal pain<br><br>Use transitions between different parts of the interview. This makes the conversation move smoothly and help the patient follow you with a clear mind without confusion. |

| | |
|---|---|
| *Have you ever had similar episodes in the past?*<br>No<br>*Have you had a medical illness or injury since your last medical check up?*<br>No, doctor. | Now ask questions using the following mnemonic:<br>PAMP HUGS FOSSED: P for Past medical history |
| *Have you ever been diagnosed with ectopic pregnancy?*<br>Ectopic? What is that?<br><br><br>*O.K, Ectopic pregnancy simple means "an out-of-place pregnancy". normally pregnancy arises inside the cavity of the womb. But sometimes, for a variety of reasons, pregnancy may develop outside the womb. It is called ectopic pregnancy. Have you ever been diagnosed with that condition?*<br>No, doctor.<br><br>*Have you ever had appendicitis?*<br>No, doctor<br><br>*Have you ever been diagnosed with pelvic inflammatory disease?*<br>Yes, doctor, when I was 26 year old I was diagnosed with PID<br><br>*Did you undergo any treatment for that?*<br>Yes, I was given some pills by my family doctor and I had relief.<br>Why are you asking about it now?<br>*That is a good question. Many current illnesses could be due to past health problems. I would like to know about them.*<br>Ok | If the patient does not understand the terms in your question, explain them clearly to the patient before you ask the question again.<br><br>Note how this doctor replaced the technical terms into the patient's language.<br>Ectopic pregnancy = out of place pregnancy<br>Uterus = womb<br><br><br><br>Appendicitis can damage the fallopian tube by causing adhesions resulting in the delay of the passage of the egg, allowing it to implant in the tube.<br><br>The history of pelvic inflammatory disease increases the risk of ectopic pregnancy |

| | Sometimes patients feel irritated by questions about their past illnesses, which they think have no bearing upon their current health problems. In such situations, patiently explain the importance of past medical history. |
|---|---|
| *Do you have any allergies, such as to medications, foods, pets, or plants?* ampicillin *What happens when you take ampicillin?* I get diarrhea | PAMP HUGS FOSSED: A for Allergies Many patients interpret side-effects of medications as allergies. Therefore, it is important to ask what exactly happens when the patient takes the medication. Often, patient had a side-effect to the medication, not allergy |
| *Are you taking any prescription medications now?* No, doctor *Are you taking any over-the-counter medications?* Yes, doctor, I have been using some vitamin tablets for energy. | PAMP HUGS FOSSED: M for Medications Patients often do not bother to inform about over-the-counter medications, vitamins, minerals etc. Remember to ask direct questions in that area. |
| *Do you have any stress in your life?* No | PAMP HUGS FOSSED: P for Psychiatric history and problems Suspect Irritable Bowel Syndrome in a patient presenting with abdominal pain and stress |
| *Have you ever been hospitalized overnight?* Yes, for pneumonia *When was that?* I guess some time 10 years ago, I am not sure | PAMP HUGS FOSSED: H for Hospitalizations Go easy with chronology of the past events. Don't grill patients to give you exact years and months. That will only frustrate them. |

| | |
|---|---|
| *Have you ever had to stay in the hospital overnight to undergo a surgery or a procedure?* Yes, I underwent tubal reconstructive surgery for my infertility | A history of tubal reconstructive surgery is a high risk factor for ectopic pregnancy |
| *Do you feel pain when you pass urine?* No | PAMP HUGS FOSSED: U for Urinary Complaints Suspect kidney stones or urinary stones or pyelonephritis in patient presenting with abdominal pain along with urinary complaints. |
| *Are you throwing up?* *No* *Are you moving your bowels regularly?* *yes* (Doctor listens attentively) | PAMP HUGS FOSSED: G for Gastrointestinal complaints Some patients do not understand the word 'vomitings'. Use layman language in such cases. Throughout the interview, beware of your body language. Avoid body movements that display boredom. |
| *Have your sleeping patterns changed in any way?* No | PAMP HUGS FOSSED: S for Sleeping History |
| *Are there any illnesses that seem to run in your family?* No *Has anyone in your family ever had anything like the symptoms you are having now?* No | PAMP HUGS FOSSED: F for Family History Family history is the exploration of the presence or absence of any disease in the patient's family which may have an impact on the diagnosis of the present illness or risk of future disease. Family history also helps in managing the illness like protecting the family members at risk in certain illnesses. |
| *How old were you when you had your first period?* 13 years. | PAMP HUGS FOSSED: O for Ob/Gyn history Obtain OB/Gy history in all female patients |

| | |
|---|---|
| *I remember you told me in the beginning that your last menstrual period was two months ago, right?*<br>Yes<br>Were *your cycles regular before?* yes<br>*Have you ever had an abortion?*<br>No<br>*Do you have children?*<br>No | |
| *Now, Mrs. Kemp, I want to ask you some questions about your sexual life. Is that all right with you?*<br>Yes, doctor.<br><br>*You told me before that you are sexual active. Do you participate in intercourse?*<br>Yes<br><br>*How many sexual partners do you have?*<br>only my husband<br><br>*Do you use any means of birth control?*<br>No<br><br>*Did you use any contraception before?*<br>I was on an IUD for four years | PAMP HUGS FOSSED: S for Sexual History<br>Use transitions when moving from one part of the interview to another.<br><br><br><br><br>The risk of PID is more in women with more than one sexual partner. Educate the patients with multiple sex partners about the risks associated with such a lifestyle Women with IUDs are four times more likely to suffer from an ectopic pregnancy |
| *Now, Mrs. Kemp, I want to ask you some questions about your personal life. Is that all right with you?*<br>Yes, doctor. | PAMP HUGS FOSSED: S for Social History<br>Social history explores about who the patient is as a person and how the patient's lifestyle influences his or her health. It also helps in planning the management of the disease, in making adjustments needed in the work schedule, in evaluating the risk factors to determine the effectiveness of preventative measures. There is always things about the patient you do not know. Since you have time constraints, limit your social history to SODA. |

| | |
|---|---|
| | S—Smoking<br>O—Occupation<br>D—Drug use & Domestic abuse<br>A—Alcohol use |
| *Do you smoke?*<br>No<br>*Did you smoke in the past?*<br>No, never | SODA: S for Smoking<br>Smoking increases the risk for miscarriage |
| *What sort of work do you do?*<br>You mean, job outside?<br>*Yes*<br>I am a housewife | SODA: O for Occupation<br>History of occupation explores the working conditions of the patient, sometimes giving vital clues to the diagnosis. For example, a plumber may have exposure to lead that leads to abdominal pain |
| *Mrs. Kemp, now I want to ask you a few questions to disclose whether you use any recreational drugs. I would like to remind you that these questions are not meant to judge your life style but rather to assist me in identifying risk factors for your illness? Is it all right with you?*<br>Go ahead, doctor<br><br>*Do you use any recreational drugs?*<br>I used to take marijuana occasionally with my friends when I was a student. But when I learnt it's bad effects on health, I rescinded that habit.<br>*Very good.*<br><br>*Now I want to ask you a question about your home life. In fact, because violence is common in women's lives, I now ask every woman in my practice about domestic violence. Has that ever happened to you?* | Use transitions whenever you move from one point of the interview to another. Also discuss their relevance before asking sensitive issues.<br><br><br><br>Make statements that praise the patient.<br>'*That's great*'<br>'*very good*'<br>'*I am glad to hear that*'. |

| | |
|---|---|
| No, doctor, we occasionally argue with each other. Never more than that | Against the backdrop of increased prevalence of domestic abuse, it is recommendable to suspect domestic violence in every woman presenting with some sort of 'pain'. |
| *Good, do you drink alcohol?*<br>No | SODA: A for Alcohol<br><br>Alcoholism is a risk factor for miscarriage |
| *Do you do any exercise?*<br>No | FOSSED—E for Exercise<br>Exercise history is an important feature of the patient profile.<br>It helps in estimating patient's physical activity |
| *"Now, tell me what you've eaten over the last 24 hours?"*<br>Just regular stuff, like pizza, sandwiches, bread | FOSSED: D for Diet<br>Exploring dietary habits of the patient helps in recommending dietary changes. (e.g. salt restriction in hypertension, sugar restriction in diabetes, saturated fats restriction in obesity, increasing fiber intake in constipation etc) and identifying any foods that act as disease causing agents |
| *Good, thank you for answering all my questions patiently. Now I would like to do physical examination on you, O.K? Is there anything else we haven't covered or that you'd like to tell me before I examine you?"*<br>*No*<br>*Any questions?*<br>*No*<br>*Excuse me for a moment, I would like to wash my hands.* | After PAMP HUGS FOSSED, do WPSCF<br>W—Washing hands<br>P—Physical examination<br>S—Summary<br>C—Closing<br>F—Farewell<br><br>Prior to starting your physical examination, wash your hands with soap. Make sure that the patient is draped.<br>Always warn the patient when you intend to do or say something unexpected or painful |

Perform the physical examination of the following:

Abdominal examination
(this patient has tenderness in the abdomen)
*"Now I am going to listen to your lungs and heart"*
*"Can you take a few deep breaths for me?"*
*"Thank you"*
Chest examination
Extremities examination (tenderness in the right shoulder)

*Now, Mrs. Kemp, let me summarize what you have informed me so far. You had your last menstrual period two months ago, right? This morning you got the sudden and severe pain in your tummy, right? You also had bleeding through vagina. Am I right so far?*

Yes, doctor
*In the physical examination, I've found you complaining of pain in your lower belly and the right shoulder.*

*So, Mrs. Kemp, based on the information you have given me and the physical examination I have done on you, I suspect a few possible causes for your condition. On the top of my list is ectopic pregnancy, that is, as I told you before, is the pregnancy that forms outside the womb.*
*Before I confirm this diagnosis, I need to run a few tests on you like ultrasonography*

WPSCF: P for Physical Examination
You don't have to be silent during physical examination. Keep talking to describe what you are doing, to reassure the patient and to gather more information you've not obtained during the history taking. Start your physical examination with areas of major concern, if you have time examine other areas of relevance

Auscultate the heart: presence of tachycardia and hypotension can be due to profuse blood loss.
Do not perform pelvic examination.
In most early ectopic pregnancies, no abnormal findings can be found.

WPSCF: S for Summary
Summarize the cardinal points of your history before starting the physical examination. Remember a summary needs to restate information that came from the patient and must have **at least 3 information elements**. In addition, summary should link various information together effectively.
Summary help the patient follow you clearly without information, report the progress of the interview and serve to check on disagreements between the doctor and the patient.

WPSCF: C for Closure
Close the encounter thoroughly by sparing a few minutes for giving a

*to rule out other possibilities like miscarriage or appendicitis. Do you have any questions for me?*

Doctor, how does the ectopic pregnancy happen?

*I appreciate your question, Mrs. Kemp, first let me give you some anatomical details of the reproductive organs so that you can understand this well. Uterus is a hollow organ or simply is the womb, to which two slender tubes called fallopian tubes are attached on both sides.*

(Doctor draws diagram of female reproductive system on the back of the scrap paper)

*Fallopian tubes carry ova from the ovaries to the uterus. After sex with a man, sperms, after being deposited in the vagina, swim up the fallopian tubes, after passing through the cervix and uterus. Fertilization occurs in the outer part of the tube near to the ovary. After fertilization, the egg normally goes back into the cavity of the womb, where it is deposited to form the embryo. Unfortunately, sometimes fallopian tubes may fail to transport the developing embryo into the womb resulting in this dangerous condition, called 'ectopic pregnancy'. The most common reason for an ectopic pregnancy is damage to the fallopian tube, causing a blockage or narrowing. In your case, you told me you had a tubal reconstructive surgery. That increases the risk of this condition. In most cases however, the cause of ectopic is not known. Am I clear to you?*

Yes, doctor, one more question: am I going to lose my baby?

*Mrs. Kemp, I understand your concern about your pregnancy. I will sit again with you to discuss how you can cope up*

summary, counseling the patient and answering the patient's questions.

**Components of the effective closing:**

1.  share your first impression to the patient
2.  do not give a definitive diagnosis, rather give a differential diagnosis
3.  explain technical terms in lay language to the patient
4.  do not give premature reassurance
5.  ask whether the patient has any questions for you
6.  address the concerns of the patient
7.  explain what you are going to do from this point
8.  end with a thank you and good bye.

Use only words of approximation even when you are definitely sure of a particular diagnosis.

Explain what is ectopic pregnancy

Inform the risks of future ectopics

Draw diagrams whenever you discuss topics which require anatomical knowledge

with this problem. I will also help you get in touch with some support groups. Right now, I need to look into your problem more carefully *through a series of tests. Then only will I be able to confidently predict the outcome of your pregnancy. When I get the lab report I would like to sit with you again to discuss the exact diagnosis and the strategies we are going to follow to bring out the most beneficial outcome. But right now, since we suspect ectopic pregnancy, you should stay in the hospital under our care Am I clear?*
Yes, doctor, thank you.
*Is there anything else you'd like to tell me or ask me?*
No, doctor thank you.

*Thank you, Good bye*

It is essential that physician always includes psychological management of the patient into his or her patient care when patient has to go through emotionally challenging situations like losing a pregnancy

Give information about local or national support groups

Close the interview with giving the patient the opportunity to have the last word

End every encounter with a thank you and good bye

# SECOND PATIENT ENCOUNTER

**64 year-old female, Martha West complaining of urinary incontinence.**
**Blood pressure = 158/90mmHg Heart Rate=88 Respiration = 16 Temperature 98.6**
**Perform a focused history and physical examination on this patient. After leaving the room, complete your patient note on the form provided.**

| | |
|---|---|
| (Doctor knocks on the door)<br>Pt: Yes, come in | Knock on the door before you enter the examination room |
| *"Hello, Good morning Mrs. West, I am Dr. Paul."*<br>Good morning, doctor | Remember the name of the patient, best way to do this is to write down the patient's last name on your scrap paper before you enter the examination room. Use the last name of the patient to address them. Do not call the patient by their first name. Tell your name while greeting them. |
| *What brings you in today, Mrs. West?*<br><br>Doctor, I am losing urine sometimes without my control. It is bothering me so much especially when I need to go to a social gathering or the church. I also stopped singing in my church choir because of this problem. | **CPR—Chief complaint**<br>Though the chief complaint is given in the doorway information sheet do not jump into the chief complaint. Start your conversation with an open-ended question. Avoid closing an open-ended question with another question. Also, avoid leading questions in the beginning of the interview. |
| *How old are you now?*<br>64 years | Urinary incontinence is most common in older patients.<br>Ask one question at a time. |
| *Please answer my questions, patiently* | History is the most important step in the evaluation of urinary incontinence. |
| *When did your problem with urine leakage begin?*<br>Almost two months ago I went to shopping with my daughter. We were busy in our shopping for about two hours; | CPR—History of present illness<br>Duration of the illness helps you decide whether the problem is acute or chronic. |

| | |
|---|---|
| Then when we had finished our shopping I tried to lift the basket in my hand. Then suddenly I leaked urine and this happened many times after that time. | Do not interrupt while the patient telling her story. Maintain pause for at least one minute.<br><br>Demonstrate genuine interest in the patient as a person, not in their illness. Respect elderly patients. |
| *What, if any thing, are you doing when you experience incontinence?*<br>when I bend over, when I cough, sometimes when I laugh, during walking, and every time I run too fast | Suspect stress incontinence in patients who complain loss of urine associated with activities which result in an increase in intra-abdominal pressure like coughing, sneezing, lifting, exercising |
| *Do you loss urine when you are not involved in these activities?*<br>No, I am perfect when I do not experience some sort of stress. | Suspect detrusor overactivity in a woman when the leakage occurs in the absence of stress maneuvers. |
| *When you need to urinate, do you experience a feeling of urgency that compels you to rush to the toilet?*<br>no, doctor | Suspect detrusor overactivity when the patient complains that her incontinence is preceded by the onset of an intense urge to urinate. |
| *How often does this type of leakage occur?*<br>About three or four times a day. I am so concerned about this problem doctor because it has not stopped.<br>*I can see you are concerned, Mrs. West.* | Address the feelings of the patient using expressions such as<br>*I can see you are concerned.*<br>*I can see you are upset*<br>*I understand* |
| *Have you noticed any change in the color of urine?*<br>No | A tumor in the bladder might show up with detrusor overactivity, leading to urinary incontinence, and hematuria. |
| *How often do you usually need to urinate during the day?*<br>3 or 4 times a day. | Establish the normal urinary frequency for the patient |
| *Does the urine flow in a good stream or interrupted spurts?*<br>It's a good stream, I guess | Suspect urethral obstruction if the patient complains dribbling. |

| | |
|---|---|
| *Do you have pain in the area of your bladder?*<br>No | Suspect urinary retention in patients who complain sense of fullness or pain in the area of bladder. |
| *Do you lose urine without warning if you are lying still?*<br>No, doctor | Stress incontinence patients do not lose urine in supine position. |
| *Do you wet the bed at night?*<br>No | |
| *Do you urinate frequently than you need in order to prevent leakage?*<br>Yes | |
| *Does any thing make your condition better?*<br>I get some relief when I do not expose myself to stressful conditions | |
| *So you have this problem for the last two months, you are involuntarily losing urine whenever you do some straining activities like lifting objects, walking or running, and you do not leak when you are lying on your bed, right?*<br>Patient nods her head | Verification help you to clarify the information you've got from the patient and give an opportunity to the patient to make any corrections. |
| *Do you have any other illnesses that have been acting up lately?*<br>Uhh<br>*Any thing like shortness of breath, palpitations etc?*<br>No, I don't think so | CPR—Review of systems<br>Ask about associated symptoms. Conditions like atrophic vaginitis are common in women who complain urinary incontinence.<br>In ROS, ask pertinent positives and negatives |
| *Were you involved in any injuries or accidents? Especially did you experience a back injury?*<br>No | Back injury might result in incontinence. |

| | |
|---|---|
| *Now, let me ask you a few questions about your past health.* | Use a transitional question when you move from one section of the history to the other. This approach helps the patient better follow you with a non-confused mind. |
| *Do you have any health problems like heart disease, lung disease etc?* <br> No | **PA**MP HUGS FOSSED <br> Exploring the the presence of past medical problems is required to assess their impact on the patient's current problem. For example, hyperglycemia in diabetes might cause excessive urine output resulting in incontinence, visual problems in a patient with glaucoma or cataract might aggravate incontinence |
| *Are you allergic to anything?* <br> I am allergic to penicillin <br> *What happens when you take penicillin?* <br> My skin will flare up | PAMP HUGS FOSSED: A for Allergies |
| *Have you used any medications to control your incontinence?* <br> No, doctor | **PAM**P HUGS FOSSED: M for Medications |
| *Are you using any medications for other reasons?* <br> No <br><br> *Are you using any pads or other protective devices to control urine leakage?* <br> No, doctor, I am just changing my underclothes more frequently | Many medications such as ACE inhibitors, alpha adrenergic blockers cause incontinence. |
| *Now, let me ask you a few questions about your mental status.* <br> *Where are you now?* <br> In the hospital <br><br> *Good, tell me today's date, day of the week, month and the year?* <br> May 20, Tuesday 2008 | PAMP HUGS FOSSED—P for Psychiatry Rule out delirium in older patients. It is the most common cause of incontinence in hospitalized patients. <br><br> Assess orientation to rule out delirium |

| | |
|---|---|
| *Have you restricted your social activities because of your incontinence?* <br> Yes, doctor, It is quite embarrassing now a days to go to church because of this incontinence. I am also worrying about the urine odor | Address this problem, which is a psychological and social impact of urinary incontinence. For many women, urinary incontinence transforms into a social stigma. |
| *Now, I want to ask you about your mental status. How have you been feeling lately? Are you feeling normal or depressed?* <br> I am feeling very well, my daughter and grandkids visiting me for summer vacation. I think this is the best time of the year for me | Depression can be a cause or complication of incontinence. |
| *Good, Have you been hospitalized lately?* <br> No | PAMP HUGS FOSSED <br> Prolonged immobility in hospitalized patients might cause incontinence. |
| *Have you undergone any surgeries like hysterectomy, or a bladder repair?* <br> No, doctor | Treatments for previous problems affecting urinary or reproductive tract have risk factors that contribute to urinary incontinence. |
| *Do you have any burning pain when you urinate?* <br> slightly | PAMP HUGS FOSSED <br> Dysuria in a patient with urinary incontinence could be the result of underlying infection of the urinary tract |
| *Do you have frequent urinary tract infections?* <br> last year I had an urinary tract infection, for which I got treatment | Symptomatic urinary tract infections commonly cause or contribute to incontinence. |
| *How often do you have a bowel movement?* <br> Every alternate day | PAMP HUGS FOSSED <br> Constipation can aggravate urinary incontinence. |

| | |
|---|---|
| *Do you have difficulty controlling your bowels?* <br><br> No | Fecal incontinence might coexist with urine incontinence, especially in patients with stool impaction. |
| *Must you strain very hard in order to have a bowel movement?* <br><br> Very infrequently | Chronic constipation may be a contributing factor to incontinence |
| *Do you have to push on the vaginal walls to have a bowel movement?* <br><br> No | Manual pressure over rectum through vaginal wall could result in weakness of pelvic muscles resulting in urinary incontinence |
| *Is your sleep affected by this loss of urine?* <br> Some times, when I get cough on my bed, I leak <br><br> *Do you wet the bed at night?* <br> No | PAMP HUGS FOSSED <br> In stress incontinence, patients do not leak in the supine position. <br> If the patient has leaks in the supine position, rule out stress incontinence and suspect total incontinence or <br> Urge incontinence or <br> Overflow incontinence |
| *Now, let me ask you a few questions about your family?* <br> Yes, doctor <br> *Does any one in your family have incontinence?* <br> No | PAMP HUGS FOSSED Family history <br><br> Use a transitional question when you move from one topic to another. |
| *Do you have any diseases like cancers running in your family?* <br> I don't know. My parents divorced when I was a teenager and I grew up with my grandma. <br> *Your parents divorced? That must have been a very upsetting event to you* <br> Yes doctor, it was | Events like parents' divorce are traumatic things in one's life. Do not ignore them or minimize them. Try to acknowledge both the facts and the patient's feelings. <br> We are living in a 'divorce generation'. Tragically, one in every two marriages end up in divorce. Many children bear the brunt of their parents' divorce and often go through psychological stress and even, depression |

| | |
|---|---|
| *Now, I want to ask you about your menstrual cycles, is that all right with you?*<br>No problem, doctor | Use a transitional question and ask for permission.<br>Do not mumble. Do not swallow your words. You should be confident in every part of the conversation about everything you say. |
| *When was your last menstrual period?*<br>about 14 years ago<br>*Are you having hot flashes?*<br>Often, I don't experience them as often as I used to but especially in the evening or at night I get up with irritation and nervousness with a craving to eat and sweating on my face and trunk. | PAMP HUGS FOSSED: O for Ob/Gyn<br>Suspect Menopausal syndrome in women, who complain hot flushes and sweating especially during hot weather |
| *Are you taking hormone replacement therapy?*<br>No, but I would like to ask you about it | The patient expressed a desire about the hormone replacement therapy. Before the conclusion of your patient encounter, you should be able to give some information about the HRT to the patient. |
| *Now, I would like to ask you a few sensitive questions about your sexual life. I know it is embarrassing to be asked about your private life, but the information you provide helps me get a bigger picture of your overall health, OK?"*<br>No problem, doctor | PAMP HUGS FOSSED<br>Before asking sensitive questions prepare the patient for the occasion by using a transitional question, explaining the necessity of questioning and the importance of the information. |
| *Are you sexually active?*<br>Yes, with my husband<br><br>*Do you experience any pain during the sexual activity?*<br>Very rarely<br><br>*Do you experience urine leakage with sexual activity?*<br>No | Suspect dyspareunia in patients who complain pain during sexual activity. |

| | |
|---|---|
| *Have you ever been diagnosed with a sexually transmitted disease?*<br>No | |
| *Now, Can you tell me a little about yourself? How have things going for you otherwise?*<br>Just normal<br>*Do you smoke?*<br>No, I never smoked in my life | PAMP HUGS FOSSED<br><br>Ask SODA in social history, S for smoking<br>Smokers cost the economy $97.6 billion a year in lost productivity and $97.6 billion in public and private health care spending. It is the responsibility of the physician to encourage the patients to stop smoking |
| *Good, what do you do for a living?*<br>I am a retired teacher. | O for occupation<br>Work related pressures lead to worsening of urinary incontinence |
| *Do you use any illegal drugs?*<br>Never, doctor | D for drugs |
| *Good, do you drink alcohol?*<br>No, never | A for alcohol |
| *Are you involved in any kind of physical activity like jogging or aerobics?*<br>No<br>*Do you know how to do Kegel exercises, squeezing the muscles to hold back urination?*<br>I never heard about them | PAMP HUGS FOSSED—E for Exercise |
| *How is your appetite?*<br>Good<br>*Do you eat adequately?*<br>Yes<br>*How much coffee do you drink per day?*<br>2-3 cups | PAMP HUGS FOSSED<br>Exploring dietary habits of the patient helps in recommending dietary changes. (e.g. salt restriction in hypertension, sugar restriction in diabetes, saturated fats restriction in obesity, increasing fiber intake in constipation etc)<br>Explore caffeine usage in patients with urinary incontinence since caffeine |

increases the urine production and worsens the incontinence

| | |
|---|---|
| *Okay Mrs.West, let me see if I have it straight. You told me that you have losing urine involuntarily for the last 2 months. This menace is particularly bothersome when you strain. Right?* (Patient nods) *The problem is gradually increasing. Right?* (Patient nods) *Now I would like to do a physical on you, then let us decide where we go from there. OK?* (Patient nods) *Excuse me for a moment, I want to wash my hands. Please untie your gown, thank you.* | Give a summary to the patient preferably before you start a physical examination. A summary is a technique by which the physician feeds back to the patient the important points of what has been said thus far. Benefits of summary: 1. Helps eliminating any misunderstandings that accrued into the communication so far in the interview 2. Helps the physician remain organized 3. Helps in the transition from one area to another area of the interview<br><br>A summary needs to restate information that came from the patient and must have at least 3 information elements. |
| Physical examination in the patient with urinary incontinence: *"I am going to untie your gown?"* *"Now I am going to do press your belly to see whether you have any abnormalities inside?"* *"Does it hurt when I touch or press?"*<br><br>9. Abdominal examination<br><br>*"Can you pull yourself all the way down to the end of the table?"*<br><br>5. *"Thank you, that's fine. Let me put this pillow under your head right there"* look for any growths, such as tumors, in the lower abdominal area. | **Preparing the patient for PE:** Drape the patient appropriately. Expose only the area you need to examine, respectfully. Explain to the patient what you are going to do Do not spend more than five minutes on physical examination Do not perform pelvic examination or breast examination.<br><br>Always start your physical examination with the areas of major concern. Otherwise, patient might think that his or her feelings being ignored or misunderstood |

| | |
|---|---|
| 6. *"What is this scar here?"*<br>7. *"I got it when my gallbladder removed"*<br>8. Palpate for bladder distention<br>9. Test for costovertebral tenderness for any urinary tract infection<br>10. Check the muscle tone in the lower abdomen<br><br>1. Check the nervous system to see if a problem is causing muscle weakness or loss of reflexes<br><br>• Auscultate heart and lungs, briefly. | Physician gathered some surgical history which patient forgot to inform in the history taking |
| *Mrs.West, it seems that you have been suffering from urine incontinence due to increased pressure in your belly, which occurs often due to stress. I am not sure of the exact diagnosis at this time. So, I need to run a few tests to determine the exact cause of your incontinence. Let's work together to get your incontinence under control.*<br>*Also, I remember you asking me about hormone replacement therapy, a while ago, do you want more information about it?*<br>Yes, doctor.<br>*Good, Hormone replacement therapy provides hormones that help menopausal symptoms like hot flashes, irregular menstruation, fat redistribution. They also help to reduce the risk of osteopenia and osteoporosis. The main hormones we give are estrogen and progesterone*<br>*Do you have any questions for me?*<br>Yes, doctor. You talked about Kegel or something exercises. What are they? | During the closure of the interview, express your collaboration with the patient using statements such as,<br>'let us work together to get your incontinence under control'<br>'we are going to plan and work to bring the best possible outcome'<br>'we', 'us' are words of collaboration.<br><br>At the end of the interview:<br>1. Share your findings with the patient<br>2. Discuss what you are going to do after this point<br>3. Answer questions of the patient<br>4. Educate the patient |

| | |
|---|---|
| *Very good question. Kegel exercises can be very helpful, particularly for urge or stress incontinence. The exercises involve repeatedly contracting the muscles many times a day to build up strength and learning to use the muscles properly in situations that cause incontinence, such as coughing. We have a physical therapist in our hospital who can teach you these exercises.* *Are you interested?* Yes doctor *Then, I will give you her contact information. All right? Any more questions?* No, doctor, thank you | |
| *Thank you, I look forward to see you again. Bye, bye.* | Close the interview with giving the patient the opportunity to ask any questions |

# THIRD PATIENT ENCOUNTER

**56 year-old Mr. John Christopher complaining of chest pain.**
**Blood pressure = 144/97 Heart Rate = 91 Respirations = 19 Temperature = 98.7**
**Perform a focused history and physical examination on this patient. After leaving the room, complete your patient note on the form provided.**

| | |
|---|---|
| Physician knocks on the door (Come, in) | Knock on the door before you enter the patient room |
| *Hello, Good morning, Mr. Christopher, I am Dr. Paul* <br> Good morning, doctor | Remember KISS <br> Knock, Introduce, Smile and Shake hand. The first thing you should do after entering the examination room is introducing yourself to the patient. Remember that a person's name is to him the sweetest and most important sound in the language. |
| *I will be your physician today and I am delighted to see you this morning, Mr. Christopher, I will be asking you a few questions about the problem, which is bothering you. First, let me put this cloth on you so that you can feel more comfortable?* <br> Thank you, doctor | Drape the patient at the beginning of the interview lest you forget to do it later. Remember KISS RED <br> R—Relax and reflect <br> E—Eye contact <br> D—Drape the patient |
| *So, what sorts of troubles have you been having?* <br> I have been going downhall for the last 3 weeks. Nothing seems to be working right. <br> *What is the worst part?* <br> My chest pain. It's gotten so bad I can't function normally. | Pay attention to your pronunciations and grammar. A good spoken English proficiency is essential to effectively communicate your thoughts and concepts to the patient. <br> Start your history using at least one open-ended question. Remember history is the most valuable tool in distinguishing the cause of chest pain. <br> Speak clearly and confidently. Check for patient's understanding frequently. |

| | |
|---|---|
| *Tell me more about your chest pains?* About 3 months ago I was mowing the lawn around our home. Suddenly I developed an uncomfortable sensation around my chest. On that day, I ignored it, thinking it was just due to a hard working day. But, this morning I got the same discomfort when I shouted at my secretary. When I informed my wife about the whole episode, she insisted me to go to the doctor, fearing it might be due to a heart related problem | Follow a logical and organized sequence to obtain the history. By asking questions, follow the problem logically starting with chief complaint, to history of present illness, then to the review of systems. Remember CPR C—Chief complaint P—History of present illness R—Review of systems |
| *In what other circumstances do you experience this pain?* Whenever I lift heavy objects or walk rapidly *How far can you walk before you get the pain?* I can walk about 3 city blocks before the pain occurs. | CPR—Probing into the history of present illness<br><br>Close-ended questions can be asked to obtain specific information from the patient. |
| *I would like to take notes of important points you tell me. Do you get the pain at rest?* Sometimes *Is the problem getting better, worse, or staying the same?* It seems to be getting worse, doctor, because sometimes I am getting the pain at rest. | Consider writing down the important positive and negative findings on your scrap paper. However, do not ask questions while looking into or writing on the scrap paper. Tell the patient that you will be taking the notes as you talk with them. |
| *Do you get the pain at night?* Yes, doctor, a week ago the pain had awakened me around 1:00 P.M and it seemed to be worse. I got up and my wife gave me a tablet. I took it and it seemed to help. This morning also I got the same kind of pain and it was resolved after 20 minutes after taking the same tablet. | Avoid linking chest pain to angina prematurely. |

| | |
|---|---|
| *Do you know the name of that tablet?*<br>No, doctor | Some people do not know the names of the drugs they use. Take it easy! |
| *OK, do you have the pain, now?*<br>No, doctor<br>*Have you ever noticed the pain after a meal?*<br>No. A meal doesn't bring on chest pain. | |
| *Have you noticed swelling of ankles or feet?*<br>No, doctor, the damn things is because my ulcer is acting up. | The amount of activity required to produce angina is usually less after meals. |
| *Does it sometimes come on while you are doing something?*<br>Yes, whenever I do things like sweeping, cleaning.<br>*How about with walking?*<br>Sometimes, when I walk faster | Suspect elevated right atrial pressures in the patients with edema in the lower extremities.<br>**"My ulcer is acting up"**: Sometimes patients interpret their symptoms and give you the diagnosis. Do not give in to temptation to accept that diagnosis. They could be wrong. Separating their interpretation from actual data is essential for an objective history taking. |
| *Now, your main problem is chest pain. Do you have other symptoms that you've had lately?*<br>No, I can't think of any. | CPR—Review of systems<br>Make a ROS only for the related systems, here respiratory, cardiac and gastrointestinal. |
| *Do you have nausea or vomiting?*<br>no, doctor<br>*Do you have cough?*<br>No<br>*Do you have shortness of breath?*<br>No | Ask one question at a time using simple short sentences<br>Pulmonary diseases like asthma, pneumonia, pneumothorax, pneumomediastinum, pulmonary embolism or pleural effusion might present with chest pain. Therefore it is necessary to ask questions related to the symptoms characteristic to those disorders<br>Ischemic pain is not related to breathing. |
| *Does the chest pain increase with breathing?*<br>No | |

| | |
|---|---|
| *Is the pain worse when you are bending?*<br>No<br>*Do you have pain in your calf muscles?*<br>No | Ischemic pain is not related to position.<br><br>Chest pain in a patient complaining of pain in the calf muscles, suspect pulmonary embolism secondary to Deep Venous Thrombosis |
| *Have you ever had racing of your heart or skipped heartbeats?*<br>on a few occasions like excitement and anger etc. | Chest pain that increases with physical exertion in a patient with a history of palpitations, suspect a *cardiac cause*. |
| *Does the chest pain appear when you press on your chest with your hand?*<br>No<br>*Do your ankles swell on you?*<br>No<br>*Are you able to lie flat in bed without becoming short of breath?*<br>Yes<br>*Do you ever wake up in the middle of the night short of breath?*<br>No | Ischemic pain is usually not elicited by chest palpation. Costochondritis and musculoskeletal disorders might present with chest pain that is elicited by palpation.<br>Orthopnea in a patient with chest pain, suspect heart failure |
| *Now, let me ask you a few more questions about your pain, show me where on the body was the pain located?*<br><br>It was under the breast bone on the left side (patient hold right fist to sternum) | Use a transitional sentence when moving from topic to topic.<br>For all pain problems ask<br>LIQOR FAAA TRIFT<br><br>Clues from location of pain:<br>Clenching a fist over the mid chest—often a clue to angina<br>"it is a sever pain between my shoulder blades came suddenly"—aortic dissection<br>"it is in my chest, jaw and the arm—myocardial infarction<br>"my chest pain gets worse with breathing"—pleuritis |
| *What is the intensity of pain, let me ask this way, on a scale of 1 to 10, where 1 is the least painful and 10 is the most* | LIQOR FAAA TRIFT<br>You can also ask, "Is it mild, moderate or severe?" to determine the intensity of pain. |

| | |
|---|---|
| *painful condition, what number would you like to assign to your pain?*<br>Probably 4 | |
| *What the pain feel like?*<br>It is difficult to find the words to describe it, doctor, it's kind of sensation of tightness, a squeezing and pressing discomfort | Quality of pain often provides clues to the diagnosis.<br>Squeezing, burning, pressing associated with exertional activities, suspect *angina pectoris*<br>It is important to recognize that many patients often do not refer to angina as 'pain' but as a sensation of squeezing, burning, pressing, tightness. |
| Doctor, I have a question, my wife always insists that cigarette smoking is a risk factor for heart disease. Is it true?<br>*I appreciate your question, Mr. Christopher, your wife is right. Cigarette smoking has been clearly identified as a risk factor for heart disease. The good news is you can decrease the risk of heart disease from abstaining from tobacco. Am I clear?*<br>Thank you, doctor. | If the patient interrupts you with asking a question answer them immediately. Do not postpone your answer. If you do not know the answer simply say that you do not know.<br>Observe how the physician has used this opportunity of being questioned by his patient not only to clarify the patient's doubt, but also to educate the patient about a risky life style.<br>Remember that SPs are specially trained to interrupt you with questions. Be ready to take the challenge! |
| *Coming back to our discussion of your chest pain, you told me that pain appeared around 1:00 pm. Does the pain in the chest ever travel to any other part of your body?*<br>Yes, doctor, three days ago I shouted on my son in the early morning for using my car without my permission. Then I got the chest pain again, and it traveled into my shoulder, arm, neck, jaw, or back. | LIQOR FAAA TRIFT: O for Onset & R for Radiation<br>Patient already told the physician about the onset of pain earlier in the conversation. So, do not repeat the question again. Repeating questions can be construed as inattention on the part of the physician<br>Most often, angina radiates to the left shoulder and upper arm, moving down the inner volar aspect of the arm to the elbow, forearm, wrist, or fingers supplied by ulnar nerve (fourth and fifth) |

| | |
|---|---|
| *Did it move into your fingers?* <br> Yes, doctor, it moved into my fourth and fifth fingers. | Diagnostic Clues from Radiation <br> Sudden, severe chest pain with radiation to the back, later progressing to the abdominal and hip areas, suspect *aortic dissection* <br> Chest pain associated with radiation of pain into fourth and fifth fingers, suspect *angina*. <br> Chest pain associated with radiation of pain into thumb and index fingers, suspect *cervical* or *thoracic disk disease*. <br><br> Prolonged chest pain for more than 30 minutes, with radiation into the left arm, occurring at rest and in the early morning, not relieved by medications, suspect *myocardial infarction*. |
| *How often did the pain occur?* <br> About 2 to 3 times per week. | LIQOR FAAA TRIFT—F for Frequency <br> Frequency reveals the severity of the disease. Interval between the attacks decreases with increase in severity of disease. <br> Diagnostic Clues from Frequency: <br> Intermittent chest pain relieved by nitroglycerin: Coronary insufficiency <br> Intermittent chest pain increased by breathing: Pleurisy <br> Constant chest pain with hemoptysis: Pulmonary embolism <br> Constant chest pain aggravated by movement: pericarditis |
| *What makes the pain worse?* <br> When I lift heavy objects, when I shout in anger, sometimes after a heavy meal. | LIQOR FAAA TRIFT <br> Angina occurs most commonly during activities like walking up hill, lifting heavy objects, eating heavy meals, during sexual activity, shouting in anger etc. |

| | |
|---|---|
| *Does coughing or moving increase your chest pain?*<br>No | Diagnostic Clues from Aggravating Factors:<br>Chest pain exacerbated by heavy meals, only on recumbency or upon bending over, suspect gastrointestinal cause—peptic ulcer, esophageal spasm, GERD etc.<br>Chest pain aggravated by coughing or moving suggests a musculoskeletal cause. |
| *What makes the pain better?*<br>Most of the times the pain goes off by itself if I just sit down and relax | Chest pain occurring with activity and is relieved by resting, suspect *angina*.<br>Diagnostic clues from alleviation factors:<br>Chest pain relief from taking antacids or baking soda, suspect gastroesophageal reflux disease.<br>Chest pain relief by sitting—inflammatory pericarditis |
| *Do you have any other complaints beside this chest pain?*<br>no, doctor | LIQOR FAAA—A for Associated Factors<br>Diagnostic Clues From Associated Factors:<br>Chest pain associated with fever and purulent sputum: pneumonia<br>Chest pain associated with hemoptysis: Pulmonary embolism |
| *Have you had any recent injuries or accidents?*<br>No<br><br>*Have you ever ingested any caustic substances like alkalis or acids?*<br>No, never<br><br><br>*Have you ever been knocked out, become unconscious, or lost your memory?*<br>No | Ask from TRIFT, T from Trauma<br><br>Rib injuries, trauma, muscle strains due to sports injuries might present with chest pain. So ask for the trauma history.<br><br>Ingestion of caustic substances—acids or alkalis—might result in caustic esophageal injury, which presents with chest pain.<br><br>Chest pain and syncope, suspect hypertrophic cardiomyopathy. |

| | |
|---|---|
| *Have you developed a rash during the course of this illness?* No *Have you developed any painful skin disease on your chest?* No | TRIFT—R for Rash Herpes zoster over the thoracic region might present with chest pain. It might present with pruritic, papular, changing to vesicular, pustular, and finally crusting rash. |
| *Did you get any infections recently?* No | TRIFT—I for Infections Infectious esophagitis might present with dysphagia, odynophagia and chest pain. |
| *Have you been running a fever?* No | TRIFT—F for Fever Pneumonia, tuberculous pericarditis, Myocardial infarction, thrombophlebitis, pulmonary embolism might present with fever and chest pain Fever and chest pain are also seen in Dressler's syndrome (postmyocardial infarction) |
| *Did you travel outside the country in recent years?* No | TRIFT—T for Travel history Traveling history explores the risk of exposure to infectious diseases like tuberculosis which may present with chest pain |
| *Mr. Christopher, now I want to ask you a few questions about your past health. You told me that your chest pain started around 3 months ago. Right? Did you have similar pain any time before that?* No, doctor | Use a transitional statement when you move from topic to topic Also, observe how the doctor used verification to clarify duration of present illness with the patient. |
| *Now, I would like to ask you about any illnesses or medical problems you've had in the past. How has your health been?* I have some blood pressure *Since how long have you been diagnosed with high blood pressure?* for the last four years | PAMP HUGS FOSSED—Past Medical Hx Past medical history exposes conditions that are causative factors of present illness Cardiac complications are the major causes of morbidity and mortality in essential hypertension. |

| | |
|---|---|
| *Are you using any medications to control your blood pressure?*<br>I take hydrochlorothiazide 25 mg daily.<br><br>*Do you have any other diseases you can think of, heart disease, or lung disease or kidney disease?*<br>As far as I know, I can't think of any | Myocardial infarction is a chronic complication of diabetes mellitus.<br>Rheumatic heart disease may present with chest pain. A history of rheumatic fever should be asked for in all patients with heart disease.<br>Valvular heart diseases, especially aortic stenosis, might present with chest pain and murmurs. Angina is one of the classic symptoms of severe aortic stenosis.<br><br>Asthma and pneumonia might present with chest pain that increases with breathing.<br>Sickle cell disease with occlusive disease might present with chest pain.<br><br>Marfan syndrome with dissecting aneurysm might present with chest pain. |
| *Now, let me ask you some other questions, Do you have any allergies, such as to medications, foods, pets, or plants?*<br>No | PAMP HUGS FOSSED, A for allergies |
| *You told me that you are taking hydrochlorothiazide 25 mg daily for high blood pressure. Are you taking any other medications?*<br>Sometimes I take an aspirin or ibuprofen for headaches and body pains | PAMP HUGS FOSSED<br>Pill-induced erosive esophagitis, most commonly due to NSAIDS, might present with chest pain |
| *How is your mood lately, are you feeling depressed?*<br>Me, depressed, no, doctor, I am living a pretty happy life with my sweet wife and two sons. | PAMP HUGS FOSSED—P for Psychiatric<br>Suspecting a psychiatric cause is also important in the patients presenting with chest pain. Patients with depression or anxiety or panic disorder might present with chest pain. For example Da Costa syndrome, which is psychogenic chest pain associated with emotional instability. |

| | |
|---|---|
| *What would you say is the thing that's worrying you the most right now?* Meeting some deadlines in my work | Remember majority of patients with depression will be seen for other complaints and may never mention depressed mood unless questioned for the symptoms. |
| *Have you ever been hospitalized overnight?* No *Have you ever been operated upon?* No *Have you ever been exposed to radiation in your chest region?* No | PAMP HUGS FOSSED Radiation pericarditis or esophagitis may present with chest pain. |
| *Are you experiencing any pain while urinating?* No, doctor | PAMP HUGS FOSSED Uremic pericarditis may present with chest pain and urinary symptoms. |
| *Do you have heartburn?* No, doctor *Have you been vomiting?* No, doctor, but . . . . (patient hesitates) *You want to say something? you don't have to feel embarassed if there is any thing that affects your health* I have been seeing some blood in my stool. *For how long?* For almost two weeks | PAMP HUGS FOSSED: G for Gastro Gastrointestinal diseases such as gastroesophageal reflux, peptic ulcer disease, gall bladder disease, foreign body in the esophagus might present with chest pain. Some patients feel embarrassed to talk about symptoms like rectal bleeding, impotence, urinary incontinence etc. Help them talk with a facilitative word. |
| *Ok, how are you sleeping now a days?* I had trouble sleeping whenever I get the pain in the night, otherwise I am sleeping well. | PAMP HUGS FOSSED: S for Sleep Angina due to coronary spasm that occurs during the night might present with chest pain. |
| *Now, I would like to ask you about your family. Does anybody have similar symptoms?* No | Family history from PAMP HUGS FOSSED Family history is not just some information you scrape off from the |

*Are your parents living?*
They are deceased

*Do you recall what they passed away from?*
My father died with cancer two weeks ago.
*I am sorry to hear that. What type of cancer?*
some belly cancer
*How old was he at that time?*
75, I guess
*How about your mother?*
She died almost 10 year ago?
*What did she pass away from?*
just natural. She died in her sleep
*How old was she?*
63
*Now, your brothers and sisters. Any history of similar problems?*
Not to my knowledge

patient as you finish up your interview. Many patients get emotional when they are reminded of their family due to issues like loss of a beloved family member, divorce, custody of a child, separation from a sibling, memories of abuse by a family member etc. Therefore, sympathize with the patient at emotional points.
Ask about the patient's parents to note for the presence of family history of premature death.(Male<55 or Female<65)
-Sometimes, emotional things like recent deaths of a family member surface in the history. Do not ignore them and move on. Make an empathic statement like *"I am sorry to hear about it" "It must have been a difficult experience to lose your mother"* etc

---

*Mr. Christopher, now I would like to ask you a few questions regarding your sexual life. That will help me to get the total picture of your health. Is that all right with you?*
Yes, doctor
*Are you sexually active?*
Yes
*Have you ever experienced chest pain during sexual activity?*
No, doctor

Follow PAMP HUGS FOSSED: S for Sexual Hx

Angina might occur during sexual activity due to coronary spasm.

---

*Now, I want to ask you a few questions about your personal life. Is that all right with you?*
Yes, doctor
*Do you smoke?*
yes, doctor

PAMP HUGS FOSSED: S for Social Hx
Ask SODA in Social history
S—Smoking
O—Occupation
D—Drugs
A—Alcohol

| | |
|---|---|
| *For how many years have you been smoking?*<br>for the last 20 years<br>*How many packs per day?*<br>roughly one pack, sometimes more than that<br>*Have you considered stopping smoking?*<br>I've tried once but I started to smoke again<br>*That's good you tried once. Don't give up. In fact, most people do not give up on smoking on their first try.* | Commend the patients who tried smoking cessation and encourage them to try again |
| *Now, tell me something about your occupation. Where do you work?*<br>I am an executive officer in the Chevron automobile factory.<br>*Is it a stressful job?*<br>Not always, but on the weekends I feel somewhat congested in my job<br>*How are your relationships with your colleagues?*<br>Pretty good relationships. But I must confess that I shout on my secretary sometimes. | O for Occupation<br><br>Competitive, aggressive and business class individuals are more prone to cardiovascular disease. |
| *Do you use any recreational drugs?*<br>No<br><br>*Did you use in the past?*<br>When I was a teenager I used to take cocaine, very rarely though<br><br><br>*Do you drink alcohol?*<br>No, doctor<br>*Did you drink in the past?*<br>No | SODA: D for Drugs<br>Ask for recreational drug use in all patients complaining of chest pain. Cocaine is associated with chest pain. It is a cause of infarction, which should be considered especially in young individuals without risk factors.<br><br>SODA: A for Alcohol<br>Alcoholism is a strong predisposing factor for Mallory-Weiss syndrome, which may present with chest pain |

| | |
|---|---|
| *Do you exercise?*<br>No, doctor. | PAMP HUGS FOSSED: E for Exercise<br>Exercise tolerance is a good indicator of severity of disorders such as dyspnea, chest pain, fatigue etc |
| *What do you usually eat?*<br>Most of the times I eat in the cafeteria in our office, which caters different kinds of foods, mostly pepperoni pizza, french fries, chicken wings etc.<br><br>*How much coffee do you drink regularly?*<br>may be one or two cups a day | PAMP HUGS FOSSED: D for Diet<br>Exploring dietary habits of the patient helps in recognizing the risk factors for many diseases and in recommending necessary dietary changes. (e.g. salt restriction in hypertension, sugar restriction in diabetes, saturated fats restriction in obesity, increasing fiber intake in constipation etc)<br>Determine caffeine usage in all patients presenting with headaches, chestpain, irritability, fatigue, lightheadedness, gastric reflux etc |
| *Well, Mr. Christopher, let me summarize what you have told me so far, you have got this pain around 3 months ago while mowing the lawn around your home, right? Often, the same pain is recurring when you lift heavy objects, right? A week ago the pain has awakened you at night, right? It is a squeezing and pressing discomfort under your breastbone on the left side sometimes moving into your left arm and jaw, Do you agree with every thing I recapped?*<br>Yes, doctor | Try to summarize the pertinent findings to the patient at least once before you start your physical examination. Remember Summary should consists of at least 3 elements of information. Summary does 3 things:<br>2.  Help the patient follow you clearly without confusion.<br>3.  Report the progress of the interview<br>4.  Serve to check on disagreements between the doctor and the patient. |
| *Good, now Mr. Christopher, I want to do a physical on you. Excuse me for a moment, I want to wash my hands.* | WPSCF: W for Washing hands<br>Wash your hands before starting physical examination. |
| **Physical examination:**<br>Perform the following:<br>3.  Observe for any xanthomas, especially around the eyes, | WPSCF: P for Physical Examination<br>Drape the patient at any time before you start physical examination. |

which are evidence of abnormal lipid metabolism.

4. Any fundoscopic changes that reflect long-standing hypertension
5. Any signs of cyanosis or clubbing
6. Inspection of precordium
7. Palpation of the heart for PMI, heaves or thrills
8. Auscultation at all four points of the precordium for heart sounds, rhythm, murmurs, rubs, gallops, clicks

I am very anxious about my heart, doctor

*"I can see that. Your heart sounds are good"*

1. Auscultation for abnormal lung sounds like rales, rhonchi, wheezing
2. Lower extremities for any signs of edema.

As little of the body should be exposed as necessary.

Always ask permission to untie the gown. To examine the upper part of the body, untie and lower the gown from shoulders. Don't lift up the gown, thus exposing the entire torso and lower extremities.

Explain what you are going to do before you do it.

After physical examination, wait until the patient is fully dressed before engaging in a conversation.

-Reassure patient if the findings are normal

Note: In many patients with ischemic heart disease, the physical examination can be entirely normal.

---

*O.K, Mr. Christopher, based on the information you have given me and the physical examination I suspect a heart problem like angina. However, I would like to take order some tests to confirm this diagnosis. For these, we would like to take some blood, urine, a picture of your lungs and an EKG. Later, you may need even a stress test.*

*Let us work together to achieve the best possible outcome. Your input is so valuable to fulfill the treatment goals of this sickness. I will gladly answer if you have any questions to ask or concerns to share with me?*

thank you, I am fine

Summary of the total patient encounter

Inform the patient that their concerns and input are valuable and necessary in order to fulfill the treatment goals.

*Before I go, I remember you telling me about smoking, right? Well, smoking has been associated with progression of this disease. You told me you tried once to stop smoking. Would like to give another try?*

Yes, doctor.

*I appreciate your decision, Mr. Christopher. First of all, let us set up a 'quit date' for you to stop your smoking completely. I will give you some literature that gives you practical guidelines on how to stop smoking. Also, I forgot to tell you, nicotine may cause migraine—that is yet another good reason to give up smoking! So, please read the literature and follow the steps. Prepare your mind strongly to quit smoking and come to my office again so that I can assess your success in that direction, OK, anything else?*

No, doctor

Counseling
The National Cancer Institute recommends the use of Four A's approach to give counseling to the patient.
Ask about smoking at the visit
Advice the patient to stop smoking
Assist the patient in stopping.
Arrange follow-up visits.

Do not give the impression that you have to run out as soon as possible, exhibit an open-ended attitude even at the end of the encounter by asking, 'is there anything else?'

WPSCF: F for Farewell

*Well, Mr. Christopher, thank you for your cooperation. I look forward to meeting you again to discuss our future course of management of this illness.*
*Good-bye*
Good-bye, doctor

# FOURTH PATIENT ENCOUNTER

**Mrs. Rachel Scott, a 36 year-old female complaining of weight gain.**
**Blood pressure = 126/84 Temperature =37.6 Heart rate=74 Respirations = 18**
**Perform a focused history and physical examination on this patient. After leaving the room, complete your patient note on the form provided.**

| | |
|---|---|
| (Physician knocking on the door)<br>Come, In<br>Physician enters into the room, well dressed, perfumed, and confident | Start your encounter with **KISS RED**.<br>Knock on the door before you enter the examination room.<br>On the day of the examination, pay attention to your hygiene. Dress in a decent professional manner. Avoid bad body odor, bad breath, dirty smelly clothing, dirty fingernails and unpolished shoes.<br>Also, remember a decent professional dressing will boost your confidence. |
| *Hello, Mrs. Scott, Good morning, I am Dr. Paul*<br>Good morning, doctor | **KISS RED:** I for Introduction<br>Introduce yourself to the patient. Do not address the female patients with words such as 'baby', 'sweetie' or 'honey'. Use only Mrs or Ms. |
| *I am glad to see you this morning, Mrs. Scott*<br>Thanks, doctor.<br><br>Doctor sits near the patient | Expressing how glad you are to see the patient that morning enhances the quality of doctor-patient communication.<br>Sit near the patient without invading their personal space. Maintain attentive posture. If you stand by the door as opposed to sit, patient may assume you are in a hurry |
| *Did you watch super-bowl last night?*<br>Yes, doctor, I enjoyed it so much<br><br>(Physician looks into her eyes and says)<br>*I could only watch the last forty minutes. I especially enjoyed Eli Manning's playing. First, let me put this cloth on you so that you can feel more comfortable. OK?* | After KISS, do RED<br>**Relax:** Talk some humor or non-medical topics and help the patient feel more comfortable with you.<br>Instead of the cross-examination approach, start your interview with talking about the sports, weather, politics, headline news, or anything non-medical. This will put the patient at ease. |

| | |
|---|---|
| Yes, doctor | **Eye contact:** Look into the eyes of the patient when you talk to her. Do not let your eyes wander across the examination room. Not looking at the patient or looking at your watch demonstrate that you are not interested in the patient<br>**Draping:** Draping helps the patient feel more comfortable and protected. |
| *So, Mrs. Scott, what brings you here today?*<br>Doctor, I have been gaining weight.<br>*Ok, I would like to ask you a series of questions about your weight gain and the other concerns, which might be bothering you.* | First do CPR!<br>C for Chief complaint |
| *Since how long have you been noticing that you are gaining weight?*<br>For the last three months.<br><br>*Are you gaining your weight slowly or rapidly?*<br>I don't know exactly whether it is slow or rapid but I'm sure that I have been gaining weight.<br><br>*Do you have any other concerns beside your weight gain?*<br>Actually, I am somewhat slowed down, doctor. I lost interest in many activities, which I used to enjoy. I am feeling irritable many times.<br><br>*(Physician leans forward)*<br>*Did any thing significant happen to you that affected you or your family?*<br>My husband was involved in a car crash about 6 months ago. Thank God, he | CPR: P for Present Illness, history of Ask about the duration of illness.<br>Avoid leading questions, like, 'you are gaining weight rapidly. Right?' Leading questions encourage the patient to tell what you want to hear.<br>Ask about the pace of illness.<br><br><br>Ask for associated symptoms.<br><br>Leaning forward towards the patient is a great way to demonstrate your interest in the patient non-verbally.<br><br>Search for a triggering event in a patient complaining symptoms suggestive of a depressive episode. Depression occurs more frequently in women than men. The presence of depression, though it is one of the |

survived the accident, but unfortunately he has been confined to the wheel chair since the accident.

*That must have been a terrible time for you and your family. I can see you are concerned about your husband. How did your husband's accident affect your life?*

Doctor, it turned my life upside down. Before the accident my husband was the sole provider for our family. Now, the responsibility of our family fell on my shoulders. (patient starts to weep)

Dt: (Handing patient a box of tissues). *Here, do you need one of these?*

Pt: thank you, doctor.

more common illnesses in our nation, is often overlooked.

Whenever a patient describes a crisis happened in their life, do two things:

First, sympathize with the patient, acknowledge their feelings and say some comforting words with a genuine concern.

Second, evaluate the effect of the triggering event on the patient's life.

Offer a tissue paper to patients who are tearful

---

*First, Mrs. Scott, we need to understand what is more bothering you right now, Your weight gain or your husband's situation?*

My husband's situation, I do not know how to run the family without his assistance.

*You told me that your husband's accident has troubled you most. What is it about this that troubles you most?*

My greatest concern is the future of my two kids. My husband's accident and his confinement to the wheel chair turned my life upside down and wrecked my life. I am feeling so anxious about our future.

I do not deserve this. I was happily married and thought I am the luckiest person in the world. I found my place in life and satisfied with it. Now, I can't believe it all came to a standstill.

*I can see and understand the disappointment and anxiety you are*

Use the words such 'we', 'our', 'us', 'you and me' as frequently as possible. These words express collaboration, which strengthens the patient and help him understand that you care about them and their situation.

Depression is extremely common in our country. Did you notice that the patient, who came to you with the complaint of weight gain, actually, had developed depressive symptoms because of a tragedy in the family? Therefore, it is essential to recognize that most patients do not come to you complaining: *I am depressed, doctor.*

Remember majority of patients with depression will come to the clinic with other complaints and may never mention depressed mood unless questioned specifically for the symptoms.

Whenever a patient complains vague somatic complaints or numerous complaints that do not fit any clear

*experiencing through this difficult time. How are you handling this situation?*
I am clueless, doctor. Everything is looking hopeless to me.
(Patient now crosses her arms and tightens her lips)

*Have you noticed any change in the presentation of your depressed mood from summer to winter?*
No change, it is staying the same all the time.

*Now, you are feeling down since your husband was involved in an accident. There are many other conditions that could cause depression. I would like to ask you a bunch of questions to identify them. Alright?*
*No problem, doctor*

*Do you get frequent headaches?*
No

*Do you have pain anywhere on your body?*
No

clinical pattern, suspect the presence of depression in such patients.
Intermittently, express empathy and understanding of the patient's concerns while continuing your interview. Remember that the genuine care is as therapeutic as offering a detailed plan of treatment.
Pay attention to the gestures of the patient. Crossing arms and tightening the lips may be signs of insecurity or anxiety.
In the patients with Seasonal Affective Disorder, patient complains that depression is more common in winter months.
Also, hyperphagia is a common symptom of this disease.

CPR: R for Review of systems
Depressed state could be secondary to physical conditions like thyroid disorders, stroke, epilepsy, metabolic disorders, cancer etc. Therefore, it is important to make an attempt to identify the symptoms of those disorders. ROS gives an opportunity to explore them.
If you want to ask a lot of questions, alert the patient with a transitive: Now, I'm going to ask you a bunch of questions I ask every body. They are very general questions and help me understand your ovearall health.
Ask questions one by one. Avoid multiple questions. Otherwise, patient wont be able to follow your questions, and you won't be able to follow his answers.
Patients with persistent headaches that do not respond to treatment might present with depression. Also, hypothalamic lesions may present with weight gain, depression and headaches.

| | |
|---|---|
| *Are you feeling excessively cold when others around you are feeling normal?*<br>No<br><br>*Are you losing your hair rapidly?*<br>No<br><br>*Do you have constipation?*<br>No<br><br>*Have you noticed your skin to be excessively dry?*<br>No<br><br>*Are you feeling excessively hot when others around you are feeling normal?*<br>No | Ask about pain in all patients you suspect having depression, because chronic pain is a common cause of depression<br>Hypothyroidism may cause mild weight gain due to edema and fat accumulation. Rule out hypothyroidism by asking relevant questions.<br><br><br><br><br><br>Hyperthyroidism may cause weight gain due to hyperphagia. Rule out hyperthyroidism by asking relevant questions. |
| *Now, let us talk about your past medical problems. How has your health been in the past?*<br>Good<br><br>*Have you ever been told that you have a heart problem, or a thyroid problem or diabetes?*<br>No, never | Now, start PAMP HUGS FOSSED<br><br>P for Past Medical History<br><br>Chronic medical problems are often associated with depressive symptoms. Beside, comorbid conditions like cancer, heart disease, thyroid problems, stroke, and diabetes may mimic depression. |
| *Do you have any allergies, such as to medications, foods, pets, or plants?*<br>No | PAMP HUGS FOSSED, A for Allergies |
| *Are you taking any medical treatment for your condition?*<br>No, I want to ask you about using medications to get out of this mess I am in right now. | PAMP HUGS FOSSED<br><br><br>Among others, reserpine, beta-blockers, alpha-methyldopa, levodopa, and estrogens are associated with depression. |

| | |
|---|---|
| *I will surely talk about it. Are you taking any prescription or over-the-counter drugs for any other illness?* <br> I am taking some vitamin tablets for energy. | |
| *Have you ever been depression before?* <br> *No* <br><br><br> *Are you feeling depressed about your current situation?* <br> I won't say that I am depressed, but my circumstances are having their toll on my life.(patient takes a long pause and talks with a low amplitude) I go to work and come back and get into my room and sleep. They show the advertisements on T.V about depressed people. But I can see all of them in me. My mind is the hell of every thing. <br><br> *You just said that your mind was the hell of everything. What do you mean by that?* <br> I think every hellish experience starts in the mind, doctor. | PAM**P** HUGS FOSSED, P for Psychiatric Hx <br><br> Patients with a history of depression episodes have an increased risk of having a subsequent attack of depression in the presence of an adverse condition. <br> Many depressed patients do not say that they are depressed. <br> About 1 out of 6 American adults have clinical depression during their lifetimes. Therefore it is essential to suspect depression in every patient who present with vague symptoms like 'fatigue', 'weakness', 'weight gain', 'weight loss', 'abdominal pain', 'loss of interest', 'unknown fear' etc. <br> Pay attention to the pauses, tone, pitch and volume of the patient's speech. In this case, frequent long pauses and low amplitude can be signs of depression. <br> **Explore the patient's clues**. It helps to understand the beliefs, ideas, concerns, fears and expectations of the patient. |
| *Now, let me ask you some questions about your sleep, appetite and other things. Have you noticed any change in your sleeping habits lately?* <br> Yes, doctor, sometimes it is very difficult for me to get the sleep. <br> *Have you lost interest in the activities, which you used to enjoy previously?* <br> Yes | Use a transitional statement when moving from one topic to another. <br> Inquire about the neurovegetative symptoms of the depression using the mnemonic, <br> **SIG-E-CAPS,** S for Sleep <br> Depression may result in insomnia, early-morning awakening, or oversleeping <br> I for Interest/ pleasure reduction |

| | |
|---|---|
| *Are you feeling guilty about anything?* Sometimes, I should have driven that day. My husband was so tired on the day of accident. | G for Guilt feelings or thoughts of worthlessness |
| *Have you noticed any fatigue or weakness during this illness?* I am feeling so weak, doctor, even the vitamin tablets are of no use. | E for Energy changes/fatigue |
| *Are you able to concentrate on the things you are involved in?* No, doctor, sometimes my mind is wandering around a million things. I am not able to help even my kids doing their homework. | C for Concentration/attention impairment |
| *Have you noticed any change in your appetite?* Yes, doctor, I think I am eating more than I used to. I am gulping lot of junk foods to reduce my anxiety. | A for Appetite/weight changes |
| *Are you feeling active or lethargic?* Sometimes I feel active and sometimes lethargic. | P for Psychomotor disturbances |
| *Do you have any thoughts or plans of hurting yourself?* Yes, doctor, many times I thought of committing suicide. But I don't want to leave my two kids motherless in this world, my boys are just 3 and 5 years old. I want to live for them, at least. -At this point patient becomes tearful and the doctor puts his hand on her shoulder, offers a tissue and says, *I understand your concerns, Mrs. Scott. Sometimes life seems too harsh. But do not lose your courage.* | S for Suicidal thoughts All patients with depression should be evaluated for suicidal risk. Five of these eight + depressed mood = Depression. Show compassion to the patients when they become emotional or tearful. Touch the patient tenderly on her shoulder as a gesture of compassion and offer a tissue. |

| | |
|---|---|
| God is testing my life, doctor.<br>*Now, do you have a plan to hurt yourself*<br>*or to commit suicide?*<br>No, I never thought that far.<br><br>*Do you have any objects in your home*<br>*like guns, pistols etc.?*<br>No | Ask about any plans to commit suicide<br><br><br>Ask about the availability of dangerous objects in the patient's home to estimate the risk of lethality. |
| *Have you ever been hospitalized for the*<br>*treatment of depression?*<br>No<br>*Have you ever consulted a psychiatrist*<br>*for any reason?*<br>No<br>*Have you ever been hospitalized for any*<br>*other reasons?*<br>The only times I stayed in the hospital overnight were for the deliveries of my two kids. | PAMP **HUGS** FOSSED<br>Ask about any previous hospitalizations. |
| *Do you have any pain with urination*<br>No<br>*Have you noticed any change in the*<br>*frequency of urination?*<br>No | U for Urologic symptoms<br>Hypothalamic lesions might present with depression, diabetes insipidus and weight gain. |
| *Some people try to reduce their weight*<br>*through induced vomiting. Did you ever*<br>*do that?*<br><br>I'm not that crazy | G for Gastrointestinal symptoms<br>Patients with depression may also have bulimia.<br><br>S for Sleep<br>Since sleep has already been asked about earlier, skip this |
| *Do you have a family history of*<br>*depression?*<br>What history?<br>*Does anyone among your parents or*<br>*relatives or any family members have*<br>*or had depression?* | FOSSED, F for Family history<br>If the patient is unable to understand your question in one way, ask the question in another way. |

| | |
|---|---|
| No<br>*Did anyone in your family attempt to commit suicide?*<br>No | Clinical depression affects the way one thinks about things and other family members.<br>Patients with a family history of depression, bipolar disease or suicide attempts are especially at risk for depression. |
| *Now let me ask you a few questions about your reproductive health. I am aware that these are sensitive questions but your answers will help me to understand your illness more completely.* | FOSSED: O for Ob/Gyn Hx<br>Use a transitional statement here<br>Slight psychological turbulence is common in a woman during major hormonal shifts (i.e. puberty, pregnancy, post-partum, peri-menopausal) |
| *You told me you have two kids, had you been able to take care of your boys after their birth?*<br>Yes | Ask about postpartum depression. |
| *Good, did you feel depressed within the weeks after the birth of your elder or younger son?*<br>My mood was slightly lower than normal. | Mild letdown of mood in the postpartum period is seen in 80% of women. |
| *Have you ever had any obsessive thoughts of harming your boys?*<br>Never | |
| *Could you be pregnant?*<br>No | Pregnancy is a common cause of weight gain. |
| *When was your last menstrual period?*<br>2 weeks ago | Polycystic ovary syndrome might present with increased weight gain associated with hirsutism and amenorrhea. |
| *Are the cycles regular?*<br>yes | |
| *Now, let me ask you about your sexual life. Are you sexually active?* | S for Sexual History<br>Patients with major depression commonly complain of sexual complaints. |

| | |
|---|---|
| No, since my husband's accident I am sexually inactive. I don't have much interest anyway. <br> *Do you use oral contraceptives for any reason?* <br> No, my husband used to wear the condoms. | Decreased sexual drive is common in depressed patients. <br><br> Weight gain is common in women taking oral contraceptives. |
| *Now, I want to ask you a few questions about your personal life. Do you smoke?* <br> Yes <br> *How many cigarettes do you smoke per day?* <br> Roughly 1 pack per day <br><br> *Since how long have you been smoking?* <br> Around 15 years. <br><br> *Have you stopped smoking recently?* <br> No <br><br> *What do you do for a living?* <br> I am a housewife. <br><br><br><br><br><br><br><br><br> *Do you take any illegal drugs like cocaine?* <br> No <br><br><br><br> *Because violence is common in woman's lives, I now ask every woman in my practice about domestic violence. Has that ever happened to you?* <br> No, doctor. | In social history ask for SODA <br><br> **S** for Smoking <br><br><br><br><br><br><br><br><br><br><br> Weight gain occurs in most patients following smoking cessation. <br><br> **O** for Occupation <br> For occupation, ask, 'Do you work outside your home?', not, 'do you work?' <br> Stressful life events in the occupation contribute significantly to the risk for depression. Discovering the mental and emotional stressors in the patient's life can give invaluable clues to the patient's state of mind <br><br> **D** for Drug abuse & Domestic violence <br> Patients with a history of substance abuse and alcohol abuse are at especially at risk for depression. Cocaine use is associated with depression. <br> Ask for domestic violence in all women, who complain 'mental' problems and vague physical complaints. Victims of |

| | |
|---|---|
| *Were you abused as a child?* <br> No | domestic violence or child abuse are more vulnerable to depressive attacks. <br><br> Patients, who were victims of abuse may become depressive in their adult life. |
| *Do you drink alcohol?* <br> No | **A** for Alcohol <br> Patients with alcohol abuse are at especially at risk for depression. |
| *Are you involved in any type of physical activity like exercise?* <br> No | **E** for Exercise <br> Physical inactivity can cause weight gain. |
| *What kind of foods do you eat?* <br> Mostly sandwiches and rice with potato and other regular foods. <br><br> *How much coffee do you drink regularly?* <br> may be one or two cups a day | **D** for Diet <br> Clinical depression affects the way a person eats. <br> Vitamin B12 deficiency and pellagra may manifest with depression. <br><br> -During periods of stress and depression, some patients drink excessive amounts of coffee and cola, resulting in other health problems |
| *Thank you for your cooperation in answering my questions, so far, Mrs. Scott, Now I want to do a physical on you. Is that all right with you? Let me wash my hands.* <br> First, do a mini-mental status examination <br> Then, a thorough physical examination is indicated to rule out organic causes of depression. Perform the physical examination of the following: <br> Thyroid palpation <br> Auscultation over heart and lungs | WPSCF—W for Washing Hands <br><br> P for Physical Examination <br> Perform the mental status examination first and then a physical examination. Physical examination is the first step in getting the appropriate treatment for clinical depression. <br> Explain what you are going to do before you do it. <br> -Asking for the patient's assistance make them feel they are not silent, inactive spectators of the process. It makes them feel as active participants of the examination. |

| | |
|---|---|
| *"I need your assistance to listen to your heart. Can you move your breast so that I can listen to your heart?"* Abdominal palpation | Make sure the patient is draped before starting the physical examination |
| *So, Mrs. Scott, let me summarize the things we have done today. You have told me that you have been gaining weight for the last 3 months. Beside you are more concerned about the welfare of your family since the accident of your husband, happened 6 months ago, right? You lost interest in the activities you used to enjoy, you are having guilty feelings about your husband's accident and there have been significant changes in your sleeping and eating habits, Am I right so far?* Yes, doctor. | WPSCF—S for Summary Note: Summary may also be done before physical examination. Make sure it contains at least 3 elements of information. |
| *Based on the information you have given, and the examination I have done I think your problems with weight gain are primarily related with unfortunate events happened to your family recently. Most probably, I suspect you have developed a depressive disorder. I need to run a few tests on your blood and urine to determine the exact cause of your weight gain and depression. I will sit with you again when the results arrive from the laboratory to discuss our future course of action to treat your illness. By the way, as a note of precaution, I want to inform you that many patients with depression commit suicide. The reasons are, most of the times, they think they are alone in their struggles. There are many groups who can offer you quality guidance to deal with your depression. Are you willing to join one of them?* | Counseling In the counseling, educate the patient about depression. Talk directly about suicide has shown to be an effective way to decrease its risk Provide the information about support groups |

| | |
|---|---|
| Ooh, no, doctor, I don't think my condition is that serious. Any way, thank you for your concern and the information.<br><br>*You are facing your problem with good courage. OK, at any time your mind compels you in the direction of suicide, call me immediately. Also, you asked me about the medications. After the tests, I will sit back with you and plan how we are going to treat this problem. Alright?*<br>Ok<br>*Do you have any questions for me?*<br>No | Recollect whether patient wanted to ask about anything during the earlier parts of the interview and discuss them<br><br>Verify with the patient whether she has any questions for you |
| *Mrs. Scott, thank you for your cooperation in the interview and the physical examination. Good bye!*<br>Good bye, doctor | WPSCF—F for Farewell.<br>Notice this patient came with a complaint of weight gain, but her real problem is depression. That came to light through careful listening to her symptoms. A common mistake is to overvalue or undervalue patient's information to suit the 'known' diagnosis. It will lead to misdiagnosis. |

# FIFTH PATIENT ENCOUNTER

Mr. David Goldstein, a 50 year-old male complaining of diarrhea
**Blood pressure = 136/89 Heart Rate = 76 Temperature = 37.8 Respirations = 17**
**Perform a focused history and physical examination on this patient. After leaving the room, complete your patient note on the form provided.**

| | |
|---|---|
| (Physician knocking on the door) <br> Come in | Start every patient encounter with KISS <br> RED <br> K for Knocking <br> Knocking on the door shows that you respect the patient's privacy. |
| *Good morning, Mr. Goldstein, I am Dr. Paul, am glad to see you this morning* <br> Thank you, doctor. | KISS—Introduce, Smile and Shake hand <br> Try to sit in a way that facilitate communication. Patient has his own 'personal space' around him. Get close enough to the patient without intruding his personal space. |
| *Mr. Goldstein, do you live in this town?* <br> No, doctor, actually I am from Pennsylvania, I have been visiting my daughter and her family for the thanksgiving. <br> *So, how was your thanksgiving day?* <br> Thanks for asking, it was very good, I enjoyed my time with my grandchildren. We had lot of turkey. Turkey for breakfast, turkey for lunch, turkey for dinner. <br> *Lot of turkey, ya, they might change the name, Thanksgiving Day into Turkey Day* <br> (Both physician and patient laughs) | *Through conversing about a non-medical topic, demonstrate interest for the patient's personal situation and everyday life.* <br> This will put the patient at ease and convince him that you are interested in the patient as a whole, not just his sickness. <br><br> KISS RED: R for Relax, E for Eye contact, and D for Draping |
| *I am glad that you had a great thanksgiving. Now, let us talk about the business, what brought you in today?* <br> Doctor, I have been suffering from diarrhea | Move your conversation from <br> General to specific <br> Casual to meaningful <br> Impersonal to personal <br> Open-ended questioning to direct questioning <br> CPR: C for Chief complaint |

*Mr.Goldstein, I will be taking some notes to record important points about your illness. Is that ok with you?*

No problem, doc

*How long have you been suffering from diarrhea?*

for the last 8 days, my wife said i must have had stomach bug, i am running to restroom, I don't know what to eat, I don't go to doctors unless I really have to, this bug or something is bothering me.

*How did they start?*

Eight days ago they started slowly, but for the last 3 days they are increased in frequency.

*Are the stools soft or watery?*

watery

*How many bowel movements do you have per day?*

Um, quite a few

*Can you tell me like, 5 times, 10 times, 15 times?*

about 10 times

*Is the diarrhea getting better, worse, or staying the same?*

I feel it is getting worse, doctor.

As you begin the interview, inform the patient of your need to take notes and the reason for it. Do not record verbatim. Limit your notes to only essential points. Your communication should look like an interview, not investigation

CPR: P for Present illness, history of

Start with a question to determine the time course of the disease. Sometimes, like this patient in our case, patients start offering etiology (e.g.stomach bug) of their problem without describing their problem. It is important to explore, 'what are the exact symptoms?' before thinking about etiology. *Avoid the temptation to think about etiology before you fully explore the symptoms of the patient.* However, that does not mean you should ignore patient's perspective on the illness.

Establish the quality of symptoms before their quanity.

Eg: how is the stool before how many stools per day?

How is the cough before how much cough per day

How is the chest pain before how many times a day

How is the vomiting before how many vomits a day

When patient describes his symptoms with vague words like 'quite a few' 'often', use more directed questions.

Patients complaining of diarrhea generally have an increase in the frequency and fluid volume of the bowel movement.

| | |
|---|---|
| *Have you noticed any blood in the stool?*<br>No<br><br>*Have you noticed any mucus in the stool?*<br>Sometimes | Frequent passage of small volume of liquid stool is common in patients presenting with inflammatory conditions or space-occupying lesions of the rectum.<br>Frequent passage of small volume of bloody stools is common in patients presenting with bacterial infection(Shigella, Campylobacter, Salmonella, and Yersinia), or ulcerative colitis, or ischemic bowel disease. |
| *What color is it?*<br>Greenish<br>*Was it foul smelling?*<br>Some nasty smell<br>*Does it float?*<br>No | F, F,F, F Stool<br>**F**rothy, **F**oul smelling, **F**loating, and the presence of recognizable **F**at droplets(oil), suspect *malabsorption.* |
| *Do you get stomach cramps?*<br><br>I sometimes get cramps below my belly button<br>(patient points his finger to the lower abdomen)<br><br>*Do you have any abdominal pain?*<br>No | You can use LIQOR FAAA for asking symptoms like pain, diarrhea, cough, fever, etc |
| *Was there any triggering event that brought your diarrhea?*<br>I cant think of any.<br><br>*Did you have any other medical disorders recently?*<br>Yes, doctor, I had pneumonia twenty days ago.<br>(Physician writes it down on his scrap paper and looks at the patient again) | As you take notes, try to look at the patient as frequently as possible. This will demonstrate interest in the person and in what he or she is saying. |

*Did you get any treatment for that?*
Yes, doctor, I have been taking Cefprozil
500 mg twice daily for the last 10 days.

*Are you taking that medication regularly
as prescribed by your doctor?*
Yes
*Have you noticed any relationship between
this medication and your diarrhea?*
I am not sure doctor, but my diarrhea started
after I started taking this antibiotic.

*Did you find out any relief method that
stops your diarrhea?*
My daughter gave me a tablet, which she
bought in CVS pharmacy.
*Uh huh*
I got some relief for an evening, but it
started again in the following morning.

Think of *antibiotic induced colitis* in all
patients presenting with diarrhea, who
have been taking antibiotics for some
other disease.

Use Facilitators To Encourage Patient
Facilitators such as silence, nodding head,
using words like *'uh huh', 'then . . . . ',
'what else?'* etc

Do not underestimate associated
symptoms. Sometimes as in this patient,
the chief complaint, diarrhea could be
due to simple viral gastroenteritis, while
the associated symptom, 'leg swelling'
could be secondary to lymphatic
obstruction by a deadly metastatic cancer
or due to deep venous thrombosis

*Now, I would like to ask you about
any ther problems that you have been
having lately. Can you think of any other
problems that you've had recently?*
I have some swelling in my right leg
*When did you first notice?*
Just a week ago
(Doctor records the point in his notes
and looks back at the patient)
*Is it painful?*
Slightly

Review of Systems
Since you are taking only a focused
history, limit your review of systems to
ones related to the present illness.
Ask the patient about general problems
first then you can focus on details of
each existing symptom.
For example, 'Do you have any
other problem I should know about?'
essentially covers ROS.

| | |
|---|---|
| *Did you remember falling? or hitting something?*<br>No, nothing sort of<br>*Ok, do you have any other problem that I should know about?*<br>No<br>*Anything like joint pains, chest pain, belly pain, pain when you pee?*<br>No | Diarrhea in the presence of joint pains, eye problems and urinary problems, suspect Reiter's Syndrome. |
| *Have you had any recent injuries or accidents?*<br>No<br>*Have you ever been knocked out or become unconscious during this illness?*<br>No | Trauma from TRIFT<br>Patients with chronic diarrhea may develop dehydration and become vulnerable to trauma and loss of consciousness. |
| *Have you ever developed a rash during the course of this illness?*<br>No | Rash from TRIFT<br>Infectious diseases like infectious mononucleosis, measles, RMSF, typhoid may present with rash and diarrhea, among other symptoms.<br>Also, drugs like ampicillin may cause side effects like rash (ampicillin rash) and diarrhea. |
| *Have you ever been tested for HIV infection?*<br>No | **Infections** from TRIFT<br>Diarrhea is very common among HIV or AIDS patients. Appropriate questions should be asked to identify the patients who are at risk of having HIV infection, because HIV-associated intestinal disorders cause diarrhea. |
| *Have you been running a fever?*<br>I am not sure, doctor, but I am feeling hotter than usual. | **Fever** from TRIFT<br>Diarrhea and fever may coexist, for example antibiotic-assoiciated colitis and many infectious diseases. |

| | |
|---|---|
| *Did you travel to any other country recently?*<br>No<br><br>*Did you go for any camping?*<br>No<br>*Did you go for fishing or hiking?*<br>I never go to fishing or hiking, but when I was young I used to go for hand gliding. I grew up in Vermont as a youngster and had lot of fun in hand gliding over the green mountains.<br>(Physician nodding his head, smiles and says)<br>*You were a hand glider, that's great, Mr. Goldstein.* | Travel from TRIFT<br>Whenever a person travels from one country to another, diarrhea is likely to develop within 2-10 days.<br>Giardiasis, which occurs among campers or hikers, may present with diarrhea.<br><br>Nonverbal cues like nodding head and smiling encourages patient to express their views fully.<br>Making sincere statements that praise the patient is one of the effective ways to improve the doctor-patient communication. |
| *Now, Mr. Goldstein, let me ask you a few questions regarding your health in the past? Is it OK with you?*<br>No problem, doctor.<br>*Do you have any heart disease or a lung disease or any other disease you can think of?*<br>No, doc<br><br>*Have you had a similar diarrhea in the past?*<br>I had diarrhea many times, but they were never this severe. They lasted one or two days and gone.<br><br>*Were you constipated for a while before this diarrhea started?*<br>No<br><br>*Have you undergone any surgeries recently?*<br>No | Past Medical History<br>A transitional statement help the patient understand the curves in your interview and follow you without confusion.<br><br>A past medical disorder or its treatment might have a relation with the present disorder<br>Helps you understand whether the disorder is altogether new or a recurrent problem<br><br>Chronic constipation may result in fecal impaction, which commonly causes diarrhea. Passage of frequent, small volume colonic fluid around the impaction may result in diarrhea.<br><br>'Postsurgical diarrhea' may occur in patients who had undergone surgeries especially, small bowel resections or gastric surgery. |

| | |
|---|---|
| *Do you have any allergies to food substances, pets, or plants?*<br>No | PAMP HUGS FOSSED, A for Allergies<br>Allergy to particular foods might cause diarrhea ( e.g. some people end up in the emergency room after having a lunch in a Chinese restaurant, due to allergy to an ingredient) |
| *Are you taking any other medications beside the antibiotic for pneumonia?*<br>No, doctor<br><br><br><br><br><br><br><br>*Have you used any medications for treating constipation?*<br>No, doctor | Medications<br>Present medical condition might be related to the medications the patient has been using. Antibiotics like *ampicillin, clindamycin, and cephalosporins* are associated with psedomembranous colitis.<br>Quinidine, magnesium-containing antacids, antihypertensives like hydralazine, reserpine, guanethidine are also common drugs that cause diarrhea. Laxative abuse is the most common cause of chronic secretory diarrhea. |
| *How are your spirits?*<br>I am in good spirits<br><br>*Do you often feel sad or depressed?*<br>No | Psychiatric condition<br>It has been observed that patients with emotional problems indulge in laxative abuse, which might result in secretory diarrhea. Therefore, it is essential to establish the emotional status of the patient and to probe into the possibility of abusing laxatives. |
| *Have you ever been hospitalized overnight?*<br>Yes, doctor, I had to stay in the hospital for 10 days when I had to get rid of pneumonia. | Hospitalizations<br>Think of pseudomembranous colitis in patients who are taking antibiotics or who had been hospitalized recently. Clostridium difficile, which is the most common organism responsible for antibiotic-associated colitis, is present in over 20% of hospitalized patients and is readily transmitted from patient to patient by hospital personnel. |

| | |
|---|---|
| *Are you experiencing pain while urinating?*<br>no, doctor | Urological Complaints<br>Diarrhea might be associated with urinary infections especially with Escherichia coli. |
| *Do you have any vomiting or nausea?*<br>No<br>*Have you noticed any change in bowel habits?*<br>No<br><br>*How often do you pass your bowels now?*<br>May be 4 times a week<br>*Have you noticed any tarry black stools?*<br>No | PAM HUGS FOSSED: G for Gastrointestinal<br>If you forget to ask this in the history of present illness, ask it now |
| *Have your sleeping patterns changed in any way?*<br>No | S for Sleep pattern changes<br>Keep an 'eye' on where you are in the interview, what you are doing and where you are going. |
| *Does any one in your family have diarrhea or vomiting etc?*<br>No<br><br>*Have you come into contact with anyone who has similar symptoms?*<br>No<br>*Does anyone in your family have belly problems?*<br>My brother had some belly cancer.<br>*What kind of belly cancer?*<br>I don't know the details. But he has some kind of belly cancer diagnosed a few years ago.<br>*Are you concerned about it?*<br>I am little bit anxious about its impact on my own health. | Family History<br>Diarrhea in many member of a family, camp or regiment may be due to a common source of infection like contaminated food or water.<br><br><br><br><br><br><br><br><br><br>The diseases of other family members often have impact on the patient's well-being. It is important to address the patient's anxieties in that area. |

| | |
|---|---|
| *Now, Mr. Goldstein, let me ask you a few sensitive questions that helps me understand your problem more comprehensively, all information you share with me will be kept confidential, is it OK with you?*<br>No problem, doctor | PAMP HUGS FOSSED, S for Sexual history<br>A transitional question helps the patient to understand where you are moving in your enquiry and keep the communication without confusion. |
| *Are you sexually active?*<br>Yes<br>*How many sex partners do you have?*<br>Only one, my wife | Patients with more than one partner are more vulnerable to sexually transmitted diseases, which might manifest with diarrhea. |
| *Have you ever had sex with another man?*<br>No, never | Men having sex with men are more prone to anal infections and thereby diarrhea |
| *Do you use any contraception during sexual intercourse?*<br>Yes, condoms | Unprotected sex is associated with various medical disorders. |
| *Now, Mr. Goldstein, now I would like ask you a few questions regarding your personal habits that give me an insight into your social life.* | Social history—SODA<br>A transitional question helps the patient to understand where you are moving in your enquiry and keep the communication clear without confusion. |
| *Do you smoke?*<br>No, never | |
| *What sort of work do you do?*<br>I work as an insurance agent in a private company. | Occupational history might give you a clue whether the patient was exposed to any hazardous or infectious material that stimulate GI tract |
| *Do you use any recreational drugs?*<br>No, never | Drug abusers are more susceptible to infectious organisms that might cause gastrointestinal problems. |
| *Do you drink alcohol?*<br>No, never | |
| *Do you do any exercise?*<br>No, doctor. Do you think it would help me at this age? | E for Exercise<br>Always answer the patient's questions. As mentioned earlier, all SP questions |

*Yes, Mr. Goldstein, it is well documented that exercise is associated with a reduced risk of heart disease. It also promotes mental well-being and protects against osteoporosis. Have you ever been told that you have problems with bones or joints that might be made worse by exercise?*
No, doctor.
*Then, you can start a moderate exercise program like brisk walking.*

are pre-programmed. You need to deal with them one way or the other. Do not skip or avoid the patient's questions.

---

*Now, Mr. Goldstein, have you noticed any association of diarrhea with the ingestion of certain foods like milk or any other products?*
No, I have been drinking gallons of milk all through my life, no problem at all! and I've not noticed any association with other foods

PAMP HUGS FOSSE**D**: D for Diet
Suspect lactase deficiency in all patients who complain of diarrhea after the consumption of milk products.
Exploring dietary habits of the patient also helps in recommending dietary changes. (e.g. salt restriction in hypertension, sugar restriction in diabetes, saturated fats restriction in obesity, increasing fiber intake in constipation etc)

---

*Well, Mr. Goldstein, I would like to do some physical examination that helps me understand more about your problem. After that, we can sit down and talk about your problems and what tests you might need"*
OK
*Excuse me for a moment, I want to wash my hands.*

WPSCF
Wash your hands with soap and do the physical examination. After physical examination, give the summary of your history taking and physical examination along with your impression of this illness and your future strategies to deal with this illness.

---

General examination for any signs of dehydration—dry mucus membranes, sunken eyes, poor skin turgor, tachycardia

Abdominal examination
Inspection: (normal)
Auscultation: (active bowel sounds)
(Physician keeps one hand over patient's shoulder and listens to his heart)

WPSCF
The physical examination in acute diarrhea is generally unremarkable, but look for any signs of dehydration.

Touching the patient empathically has a great therapeutic effect. It has symbolic value that connects the physician with the patient

| | |
|---|---|
| Percussion: (normal)<br>Palpation:(mild left lower quadrant tenderness is found in this patient)<br>Examination of right leg | Because patient complained of right leg pain, it is important to examine that extremity |
| *All right, Mr. Goldstein, now let me summarize to you what I have been considering so far. You told me that you have been suffering from diarrhea for the last 8 days, right? You also told me that you have had pneumonia twenty days ago for which you have been taking antibiotics. Right?*<br>*Now, Mr. Goldstein, many patients on antibiotics, particularly the one you have been taking, develop antibiotic associated colitis, which often present with diarrhea of this kind. In the physical examination I have found that you there are some sensitive areas over your abdomen. I suppose that your diarrhea might be related to the using of antibiotics. But there are also other causes for diarrhea like infections. I am not exactly sure what might be the underlying cause of your illness at this time, hence I would like to carry out a few diagnostic tests that will help me to come to a definitive diagnosis of your illness. Also, your right leg pain might be due to a simple muscle twitch and there are many other things that could cause sweeling and pain in the leg. I will run a scanning test to rule out any serious problems like a blood clot.*<br>*Meanwhile, I want to inform you that many patients with diarrhea lose lot of fluids from their body get dehydrated. So, I encourage you to drink plenty of fluids. Alright?*<br>Ok | WPSCF<br>Two benefits of summary:<br>1.  it helps the patient to follow your guidance more effectively.<br>2.  it helps you to make sure that you have obtained the accurate and pertinent information from the patient, on which you are going to base your diagnostic impressions and diagnostic work-up.<br><br>Counseling from WPSCF<br>Patient should be taught on how to prevent dehydration. |

| | |
|---|---|
| *I will gladly answer if you have any questions or doubts regarding your illness . . .*<br>I have no questions, thank you, doctor.<br>*Thank you, bye, bye* | Verify whether patient has any questions for you. You should exhibit a open-ended attitude even at the end of the interview. Do not give the impression that you got to run out as soon as possible<br>Farewell from WPSCF<br>Close your interview with a pleasant smile added with a thank you and good bye |

# SIXTH PATIENT ENCOUNTER

Mr. Daniel Harvey, a 63 year-old male with history of diabetes; new to your practice; came to your clinic for medication refill

Blood pressure = 138/89 Heart Rate=83 Respirations = 19 Temperature = 98.7

| | |
|---|---|
| *(Physician knocks on the door)*<br>Come in<br>*Hello, I am Dr.Paul; are you Mr. Harvey?*<br>Yes<br>*Nice to meet you, Mr.Harvey. How are you doing today?*<br>I am doing fine. How about you?<br>*I am doing great. I'll be the physician today and I am here to help you. I want to cover you with this cloth so that you can feel more comfortable. Is that all right with you?*<br>Yes, doctor. | Start with KISS<br>Knock, Introduce yourself, Smile and Shake the patient's hand.<br><br>RED<br>Relax, maintain Eye contact and Drape.<br><br>Pay attention to the patient throughout the encounter. Patients want to feel that they have your undivided attention and care. Do not rush the patient. |
| *So, how can I help you this morning, Mr. Harvey?*<br>I have been using medications for my diabetes. I need a refill.<br><br>*Are you taking your medications regularly?*<br>Yes, doctor | CPR—Chief complaint<br>Two blood glucose levels greater than 125mg% fasting or greater than 200mg% 2 hours post glucose load are defined as diabetes. |
| *I appreciate that you are taking your medications regularly and coming for a refill this morning. Because Diabetes is a disease that affects almost every organ in the human body, we should make sure that various organs in your body are functioning well while you are taking medications to control the disease. To fulfill that task, I need to ask you a series of questions and do a physical examination on you. Is that all right with you?*<br>Yes, doctor | Making statements that praise the patient is one of the most effective ways to enhance patient compliance.<br>Explain to the patient why the history taking and physical examination are essential even in the visit for a drug refill. |

| | |
|---|---|
| *Do you have any complaints now?* Doctor, sometimes I am becoming excessively thirsty. I need to go to restroom so often that I am becoming sick of this life. | CPR—History of present complaint Many patients with type 2 diabetes present with increased urination and thirst. |
| *When were you diagnosed with diabetes?* Fourteen years ago. | People with diabetes have a high risk of developing eye, kidney, foot, nerve, cardiac, and vascular complications. |
| *Type 1 or type 2?* Type 2 | There are 3 main types of diabetes: Type 1, Type 2, and Gestational diabetes, which occurs during pregnancy. About 95 percent of people with diabetes have type 2 diabetes. It usually begins after age 40. |
| *What problems you got fourteen years ago that led to the diagnosis of diabetes?* Actually, doctor, I was not aware of my diabetes for a long time. I started to drink too much water and eat too much and was constantly on a hunt for sweets. They found it out in a routine laboratory examination. | |
| *How did you manage your diabetes?* It started as a mild case controlled by diet and exercise and has progressed to oral medication for the last 4 months. | |
| *How was your health during the last fourteen years?* I am doing pretty O.K. except some skin infections now and then. Also, doctor, I am feeling tired all the time. | Chronic skin infections are common in diabetes. |
| *How is your vision?* Pretty good, doctor | |
| *Do you have any blurring or clouding of your vision?* | CPR—Review of systems In people who have had diabetes for 10 years or longer, nearly half have some degree of diabetic retinopathy. |

No, my vision is all right, but my previous doctor insists that I get my eyes checked annually. Is this really necessary?

*Yes, regular eye examinations for people with diabetes are so important because diabetic eye disease may occur as a complication of diabetes. In fact, diabetic retinopathy is a leading cause of blindness in America today. Unfortunately, often there are no symptoms in the early stages of disease. Vision may not change until the disease becomes severe. That is why we need to examine your eyes annually to detect any changes that represent diabetic eye disease. Am I clear to you?*

Yes, thank you, doctor.

*You're welcome, now, have you lost any weight?*

No

*Are you feeling any numbness or burning pain in your hands or feet?*

Yes, doctor, for the last 3 months my hands and arms feel like they are asleep while I am using them.

*How do you feel in your hands?*

It's a burning, tingling feeling and no matter how much I shake them, that feeling doesn't go away for a while. Sometimes I put an ice pack on my feet. It gives me some relief.

*Do you have chest pain?*

No

*Do you have any shortness of breath?*

No

ROS can also be done during physical examination. For example, when you examine the eyes with ophthalmoscope, you might ask whether patient has any problems with vision

Learn to be a good listener. Active listener listens with his mind and responds both verbally and physically.

Frequent use of courteous phrases like 'thank you', 'you're welcome' cements the formation of rapport between the doctor and patient.

Peripheral vascular disease may present with intermittent claudication, which is leg pain on walking or exercising that stops quickly with rest.

Diabetic radiculopathy present with pain in the front of the thigh, chest, back or pelvis.

| | |
|---|---|
| *Are you experiencing any cramps in your legs while walking?*<br>No | Diabetic neuropathy may affect the lower legs and feet causing numbness, tingling, sharp or burning pain, cramps and hypersensitivity. Diabetes is the number one cause of lower limb amputations in the United States. |
| *Do you have any ulcers on your feet or infections that are not healing with drugs?*<br>No | Individuals with diabetes are at increased risk of cardiovascular disease caused by atherosclerosis, which may result in coronary artery disease, cerebrovascular disease, and peripheral vascular disease. Think of claudication in the patients complaining of pain in the back of their legs when walking.<br>Peripheral neuropathy combined with peripheral vascular disease can develop foot ulcers and infections, which can lead to gangrene and amputations. |
| | After CPR, ask<br>TRIFT PAMP HUGS FOSSED |
| *Have you had any recent injuries or accidents?*<br>No | Wound healing is delayed in individuals with diabetes. |
| *Have you ever been knocked out, become unconscious, or developed sweating, tremors, or tingling in the hands and feet?*<br>No | Ask about hypoglycemic attacks in all individuals with diabetes. Symptoms of hypoglycemia may include sweating, dizziness, trembling, hunger, confusion, seizures and loss of consciousness. |
| *Have you ever been told that you got hypoglycemia or ketoacidosis? Or let me ask this way, have you ever developed attacks with sweating, anxiety, irritability, blurred vision, hunger, pallor, tingling lips and palpitations?* | All patients with diabetes should be asked whether they have had ketoacidosis, hypoglycemia or infections and with what frequency. |
| So far I am O.K. doctor, but what shall I do to prevent hypoglycemic attacks? | The patient education is done throughout the encounter. When the patient asks a |

*That is a very good question, Mr. Harvey. People on treatment for diabetes are always at the risk of hypoglycemia. So, at all times carry some glucose snacks with you to treat hypoglycemia symptoms. Also wear a diabetes identification card which will help prompt the people to assist you in case if you are found unconscious. Am I clear?*

Yes, Doctor, I've heard about this new pill, Januvia. Does it cause abdominal pain?

*To be honest, I don't know, but I can verify about it and tell you later.*

question, use that opportunity to educate the patient. Equally important is the fact that you should answer the patient, no matter how you feel about it, because the standardized patients ask you the questions purposefully and they use their checklist to note whether you have answered their questions or not.

Genuineness, beside respect and empathy, enhances communication between the physician and the patient. Always respond genuinely when patient asks questions beyond your knowledge or expertise. If you don't know, do not hesitate to say, 'I don't know'

| | |
|---|---|
| *Have you ever developed a rash during the course of this illness?*<br>No | Rash from TRIFT<br>In diabetics, rash with itching is common in the genital areas caused by fungal infections of glucose-rich urine. |
| *Have you been diagnosed with any skin or dental infections?*<br>No<br><br>*Do you have itching anywhere on your body?*<br>No | Infections from TRIFT<br>Ask for prior or current infections, especially foot problems, TB, recurrent urinary tract infections, skin, and dental infections.<br>All individuals with poorly controlled diabetes are at increased risk for infections, especially infections of skin and vagina. Acanthosis nigricans is frequently found in people with diabetes. |
| *Have you been running a fever?*<br>No | **Fever** from TRIFT |
| *Do you travel frequently?*<br>I go to Danville in the weekends to see my grandkids. Otherwise, not much. | **Travel** from TRIFT<br>Individuals with diabetes, who travel more should be instructed to take more |

| | precautions to prevent hypoglycemic attacks. |
|---|---|
| *Now, I want to ask you a few questions about your past medical health. Tell me about any serious illnesses you have had in the past, starting from when you were a child*<br>No problem, doctor. Yes, I had prostate cancer 4 years ago. I had 16 radiations so far to treat that condition. Now, at last I am cancer free. | PAMP HUGS FOSSED WPSCF, P for Past Medical History<br>In the past medical history, ask for the history of any acute complications like hypoglycemia, ketosis, including frequency, severity, and cause, presence of hypertension, heart disorder, lipid disorders and thyroid disorders. |
| *Were you able to cope up with that illness?*<br>By the grace of God, I recuperated well. I was exposed to Agent Orange in Vietnam. That might be the reason for my prostate cancer. I don't know.<br>*I am sorry to hear that Mr. Harvey, have you had a medical illness since your last check up?*<br>Yes, I had a kidney stone 6 months ago treated with ESWL<br>*Were you ever operated on, even as a child?*<br>No | Patients with type 1 diabetes have an increased frequency of autoimmune disorders, especially thyroid disease.<br>**Practical Point**: Focus on what being said by the patient rather than their mannerisms or physical characteristics. When patients say sad things, respond with sympathy while demonstrating your interest in the patient as a person and not like a history-taking machine.<br><br>As you listen to the patient, focus on their voice and compare their voice with the patient's body language and words. |
| *Now let me ask you a few questions about your allergies and medications? OK?*<br>*Do you have any allergies, such as to medications, foods, pets, or plants?*<br>No | **Allergies** from PAMP HUGS FOSSED |
| *What are the medications you are taking for diabetes?*<br>Glucophage 500mg tablet 3 times a day.<br>Micronase 5 mg tablet 2 time a day. | Medications<br>Ask about the side-effects of anti-diabetic drugs. |

*Have you been having any nausea, vomiting, or diarrhea after taking Glucophage?*
Yes, doctor, sometimes I am having vomiting and diarrhea after taking this drug.
*How are you dealing with those problems?*
They are stopping on their own.
*OK, are you gaining weight or losing weight?*
It seems I am gaining a few pounds, doctor.

Metformin (Glucophage) has gastrointestinal side effects like anorexia, nausea, vomiting, diarrhea and abdominal discomfort.

The major side effects of sulfonylureas are hypoglycemia and weight gain.

*You came for a drug refill for the treatment of diabetes. Are you taking any other medications for other purposes?*
I take a zolpidem tablet occasionally for sleep.
*Are you monitoring your glucose level at home?*
Yes, doctor
*How are the values showing?*
They are pretty normal

Ask for whether the patient has been using any other medications

Ask for self-monitoring

*How are your spirits? Do you often feel depressed or sad?*

Doctor, I feel depressed sometimes when I remember the horrible deaths of my friends in our cavalry who fought in the Vietnam war front along with me. You could not even imagine how horrible I have been feeling these last several months when the war memories creep into my mind. I escaped death some 19 times in a hair's breadth.

PAMP HUGS FOSSED: P for Psych Hx
Since depression became a wide spread disease in our culture, it is wise to ask every patient, especially one with chronic illnesses or past military service, about his mental status.

Suspect Posttraumatic Stress Disorder in all war veterans, police officers and people involved in accidents or any other disturbance.

Even when the patient treks on a long road of explanation, let him move smoothly, do not interrupt. It has been

*Have you contemplated committing suicide recently?*
No, doctor, I believe in God and get strength from reading my Bible. I never thought of committing suicide.

*Are you taking any medications for that?*
No

proved, that doctors who interrupt their patients do not benefit much.

Remember patients want enough time to tell their story, to be listened to, and to be cared for as individuals. Interrupting the patient is a sign of impatience or even, carelessness.

Do not criticize a patient's religious beliefs even if they sound 'unscientific' to you.

Do not insist medical treatment if the patient has other ways to cope up with his depressive attacks.

---

*Have you ever been hospitalized overnight?*
Oh, many, many times.
*When was the last time you were hospitalized?*
Six months ago when I was treated for my kidney stones.
Doctor, I want to tell you one thing. Is it OK?
*Yes, go ahead.*
You are very nice to me. Thank you for that. Six months ago, I joined in this hospital for the treatment of kidney stones. One evening I was in pain and moaning and groaning in my bed. One young doctor—I don't know his name but everybody calling him a 'fellow'—came to my bedside and shouted at me, *"Be silent. Why are you moaning and groaning?"* It hurt me a lot. I thought that doctor would understand my pain only if he had a kidney stone in his loin.

*I am sorry to hear that Mr. Harvey. I wish it were never happen.*

PAMP HUGS FOSSED: H for Hospitalization
History of hospitalizations may help you discover the presence of any diseases, emergencies, treatments and surgeries the patient experienced previously.

Patients carry the memories of their hospitalizations a long way than we think. Their current interactions with the medical staff are being influenced by their previous experiences with the hospital staff. Give an opportunity to the patient to vent off their feelings.

Remember every harsh word or rude manner will be etched in the memory of the patient to cripple him or her for a long time.

Sympathize with the patient and express your agreement with the patient when they

| | |
|---|---|
| | recount their bad experiences, especially which occurred in medical settings. |
| *Now, let me ask you some more questions about your overall health. Are you experiencing pain while urinating?* No *Are you finding it difficult to empty your bladder while urinating?* No *Are you finding it difficult sometimes to hold your urine or are you wetting yourself?* No | U for Urinary complaints Autonomic neuropathy seen in some individuals with diabetes may present with urinary incontinence and difficulty emptying the bladder. Adopt a proper body language for every patient encounter. Avoid inappropriate gestures. |
| *Do you have any complaints related to your digestive system like nausea or vomiting?* Yes, doctor, I am feeling heart burn sometimes after a heavy meal. *How do you get relief when you get heart burn?* I take an antacid and it goes away. *Are you opening your bowels regularly?* Yes, doctor. *Do you have any other complaints related to your digestive system?* No | G for Gastrointestinal complaints Autonomic neuropathy seen in some individuals with diabetes may present with difficulty swallowing, nausea, vomiting, constipation, diarrhea, dizziness and lightheadedness. Avoid fiddling with your stethoscope, pen, eyeglasses, tuning fork, paper, reflex hammer or any other instrument during your conversation with the patient. |
| *How are you sleeping these days?* Sometimes I get the flashes of my combat in Vietnam and it disturbs my sleep. Otherwise, pretty good. | S for Sleep |
| *Now, a bit about your family, are there any illnesses that run in your family?* On my father's side there is a long history of diabetes. My father, grandfather, grandmother and uncle all have or have had it. *Any other diseases beside diabetes?* No | FOSSED: F for Family history Mostly, development of type 2 tends to run in families. |

| | |
|---|---|
| *Now, I would like to ask you a few questions regarding your sexual life. Is it O.K with you?*<br>Yes, doctor.<br>*Are you sexually active?*<br>Yes<br>*Do you participate in intercourse?*<br>Yes<br>*Do you have any problems with erection?*<br>No | S for Sexual history<br>Use transitional statements at all curves of the interview.<br>Though absent in this patient, impotence is common among individuals with diabetes.<br><br>Learn to do everything confidently. Avoid communicating the words or body movements of indecision to the patient. E.g. sentences like *When was the last time you . . . uhhhhh, don't mind* or actions like opening and closing mouth without saying anything. |
| *Now, I want to ask you a few questions about your personal life.Do you smoke?*<br>No<br>*Did you smoke before?*<br>Never<br>*Good* | SODA in Social History<br>S for Smoking<br>Smoking, hypertension, dyslipidemia, obesity are risk factors for atherosclerosis. |
| *What do you do for a living?*<br>I am a Vietnam veteran. | O for Occupation<br><br>Avoid licking, wetting, pursing or biting your lips during your conversation with the patient. |
| *Good, do you use any illegal drugs?*<br>No, doctor, never<br>*Do you drink alcohol?*<br>No | D for Drugs<br>Avoid biting or chewing nails as you talk to the patient. |
| *Did you drink alcohol?*<br>I used to. But I cut it down now.<br><br>*Did you drink a lot before?*<br>No, just occasionally | A for Alcohol<br><br>Do not judge a patient's lifestyle. Avoid making offensive, insensitive, or rude statements. |

| | |
|---|---|
| | Never make comments that insult patient's racial or religious or regional background.<br><br>Frame questions objectively. Remove any preconceptions from your questioning. |
| *Are you involved in any type of physical activity like exercise now?*<br>No | PAMP HUGS FOSSED: E for Exercise<br>In diabetic patients, as in others, exercise increases cardiovascular fitness, helps to maintain ideal body weight, gives a sense of mastery in daily activities and complements dietary compliance. |
| *Are you taking any special diet for your diabetes as directed by the nutritionist?*<br>Yes, doctor, but sometimes I have such a craving for chocolate, it drives me bonkers. I don't like taking artificial sweeteners. Also, sometimes, I experience excessive sweating when I eat. They I will get clammy and sweaty.<br>*That could be due to the effect of diabetes on your nerves*<br>Ok | FOSSED, D for Diet<br>In most individuals with type 2 diabetes, treatment begins with weight reduction through diet and exercise.<br>Some people with diabetes do get sweating whey they eat, called gustatory sweating. This is due to neuropathy of the autonomic system. |
| *Thanks for answering all my questions, now I would like to wash my hands and do a physical on you. Now, Mr. Harvey, I am aware that you stepped into my office just for a drug refill. But I need to examine your eyes, heart and feet. Why do I want to check your body now? Because diabetes may involve your blood vessels, nerves, skin and lens of your eyes, leading to complications that involve many organs of your body, most commonly heart, brain, kidney, legs, and eyes. Diabetic eye disease, for example, is the leading cause of new blindness among adults in our nation. The good news is we can prevent* | WPSCF<br>Washing hands and Physical Examination |

*many of the complications of diabetes by examining your body periodically and taking appropriate preventive measures. So, I want to do a thorough physical examination on your eyes, heart, skin, and legs to check for any changes that represent a disease process. Is that all right with you?*

Yes, doctor.

PHYSICAL EXAMINATION
Fundoscopy for signs of diabetic retinopathy
Tests for visual acuity
Oral examination
Thyroid palpation
Chest and heart auscultation
Lower extremity examination
Foot inspection
Skin examination
Nails
Pulses
Sensation

Explain the importance of physical examination to this patient, who came just for a drug-refill.

---

*Ok, let me summarize the main things. You have come for a medical refill for the treatment of your diabetes; you are doing well except heart burns after a heavy meal, and sleep problems when the memories of your Vietnam combat come into your mind, right?*

Yes, doctor.

WPSCF: S for Summarization

---

*I have some possibilities in my mind. One is you can be having diabetic gastroparesis, which is a disease affecting your esophagus and the other being posttraumatic stress disorder which is a disease that occurs in individuals exposed to extremely stressful conditions like accidents, and in your case a war.*

101

*I would like to take some tests to assess the controlling of diabetes. For these I would like to take some blood and urine. Meanwhile, I will write a prescription for a refill. Use the same drugs you have been using taking the same precautions. When the results of the lab tests arrive, I would like to sit with you again and discuss what we are going to do with these problems. Before, I go, do you have some questions for me?*

WPSCF: C for Counseling

Yes, doctor, what can I do to help control my diabetes?
*That is a very good question. First, learn as much as you can about diabetes. We have a diabetic education class in our hospital, conducted every Monday and Friday 4:00 PM to 5:00PM. I encourage you to attend this class, which gives you a lot of information about diabetes. Check and record your blood sugar levels regularly at home. You can delay or prevent late complications like retinopathy, neuropathy, nephropathy by keeping tight control of your blood sugar. On your every visit to my office please bring the record book of your blood sugar levels.*
*Eat healthy food and control your weight. Take the medications as I directed. Wash your feet everyday and check them for cuts, sores or swellings. If you notice any insensitive areas on your feet, visit me immediately. Never go barefoot; wear soft clean socks and well-fitting shoes. If you develop any calluses or warts on your feet never try to remove them by yourself. Always show them to me. Also, you should take care of your eyes, gums and teeth by visiting your eye doctor and dentist regularly. You can lower your risk of heart*

| | |
|---|---|
| *disease by eliminating any risk factors for atherosclerosis, such as high blood pressure, high blood levels of cholesterol, cigarette smoking and obesity. Also, I recommend you to take influenza and pneumococcal vaccine shots to prevent those diseases.*<br><br>*I remember you told me that some of your war memories are still haunting you sometimes. Right? There are many organizations especially formed by the Vietnam veterans to assist people like you. I will be glad to give you their phone numbers if you are willing to join them?*<br><br>Yes, doctor.<br><br>*Call 1-800-VIETVET*<br><br>*Or you can also visit their web site, www.vietnamveterans.com* | |
| *Do you have any questions for me?*<br><br>No, thank you, doctor<br><br>*Thank you, good-bye.* | F for Farewell |

# SEVENTH PATIENT ENCOUNTER

Mr. Thomas Bell, a 26 year-old male wish to undertake SCUBA Diving. He is required to submit a completed medical form signed by a physician. Take appropriate medical history, perform the tasks listed on the form and sign it.

| | |
|---|---|
| *Hello, Mr. Bell, I am Dr. Paul. How are you doing this morning?*<br>I am fine, thank you. Doctor, I want to undertake SCUBA Diving starting this December. Could you please examine me and fill this examination form? (Mr. Bell hands out the examination form to Dr. Paul)<br><br>*Sure, Mr. Bell, I am glad to know that you are going to learn SCUBA diving. First of all I need ask you a series of questions to decide your health status. Is that all right with you?*<br>Yes, doctor | As usual, start your patient encounter with KISS RED<br><br>For all patient who come for pre-employment check-up or insurance check-up, do four things.<br>1. Do ROS and TRIFT<br>2. Evaluate the fitness of patient's health against the demands of the job or the program they are going into.<br>3. Ask PAMP HUGS FOSSED<br>4. Do all the things asked for on the form |
| *Now, I would like to ask you about any problems you've had recently?*<br>*Have you ever experienced dizziness or fainting?*<br>No, doctor<br><br>*Do you wear glasses or contact lenses?*<br>No<br>*Do you have persistent headaches?*<br>No<br><br>*Have you ever experienced seizures?*<br>No<br><br>*Have you ever experienced loss of consciousness during the last five years?*<br>No | For all 'fitness' forms or pre-employment application forms, make a review of systems. Think in the 'head-to-toe' approach to remember the things to ask about, asking important questions about each system<br><br>Develop good communication skills. In a study, 71% of patient cited poor communication and relationships as a reason for their malpractice suits<br><br>Speak with lively, not lazy, lips.<br><br>Since you are dealing with a complete stranger in Clinical Skills test, it is better to speak a little more slowly than your regular pace. |

| | |
|---|---|
| *Have you ever had any sinus troubles?*<br>No | Ask one question at a time, don't chop your talk into jerky fragments. |
| *Do you have any ear troubles?*<br>No<br><br>*How is your hearing?*<br>Good<br>*In both ears?*<br>Yah<br><br>*Do you develop shortness of breath with efforts like stair climbing or brisk walking?*<br>*No*<br><br>*Do you have persistent coughs?*<br>No<br><br>*Do you have severe or frequent colds?*<br>No | Serious ear problems like chronic middle or inner ear infections, Meniere's disease, and permanent perforation of tympanic membrane should prohibit scuba diving. Underwater diving propels a great barometric stress to the ear. Tympanic membrane perforation is an absolute contraindication to diving.<br>Individuals with only one hearing air should be discouraged from SCUBA because of the risk of ear injury.<br>If the applicant complains of shortness of breath with simple efforts like stair climbing or brisk walking, he is probably physically unfit for scuba diving.<br><br>Be courteous in speaking with the patient.<br><br>Individuals with persistent upper respiratory infections should be discouraged from diving. |
| *Have you ever had a serious injury?*<br>No<br>*(Physician maintains a clear voice and asks)*<br>*Were you ever involved in an accident?*<br>No<br>*Have you ever knocked out, become unconscious, or lost your memory?*<br>No | TRIFT, T for Trauma<br><br>Do not whisper |
| *Have you ever developed a fever with rash?*<br>No | Rash<br>Ask closed-ended questions to obtain specific information, but avoid leading questions. |

| | |
|---|---|
| *Have you ever had repeated infections?* No *Have you ever been tested for HIV infection?* Yes, it was negative | Infections History of repeated infections may a clue to investigate for a disorder of immunity. HIV infection is not a contraindication for scuba diving. In fact, studies have shown that sports participation benefit the HIV/AIDS patient both mentally and physically. |
| *Have you been running a fever?* No *Have you ever had hay fever?* No | Fever Do not ask multiple choice questions. |
| *Now, tell me about any diseases you have had in the past, starting from when you were a child?* I don't have any | Past medical history Use transitional statements while moving form one topic to another. Diabetes that requires insulin, epilepsy that requires drugs to prevent seizures, history of spontaneous pneumothorax, bullous lung disease, asthma that requires drug treatment for prevention of symptoms should prohibit diving. |
| *Have you underwent any surgeries before?* No | History of otosclerotic surgery should prohibit diving. |
| *Do you have any allergies for drugs?* I am allergic to Neomycin. *What kind of reaction did you have to that drug?* I got a rash *Have you had to be hospitalized for this allergy?* No, It went off by its self. *Do you have any allergy to stinging insects?* No | Allergies Individuals with persistent allergies should be discouraged from diving. Avoid medical jargon while talking to the patient. In fact, those 'big words' you use might hamper the flow of communication. Patient might also think that you are trying to prove your superiority to him, by using medical terminology. |

| | |
|---|---|
| *Now, I want to ask you about your medications. Are you using any regular medications?* I take Ibuprofen for headaches, sometimes. | PAMP HUGS FOSSED, M for Medications |
| *Any medications over the counter?* No, Doctor, I just want to know, why are you asking all these questions? I have come here just for a signature on that form? *That's a good question, Mr. Bell, but it is very important that I ask you about your past medical history and medication history. Because I must rule out whether you have any diseases, which make you vulnerable to potential dangers if you involve in SCUBA diving, I need to ask all these questions. Am I clear to you?* Yes, thank you, doctor. (Physician maintains a good posture throughout the interview) | Explain difficult or potentially confusing words to the patient. Not all SPs are nice patients. Some of them will be instructed to display seductive or aggressive or dependent attitudes towards the doctor Never get angry with the patient, even if they are aggressive, but answer their questions, patiently and clearly. For a good posture, do not cross your legs, but place your feet squarely on the floor to distribute your weight evenly. |
| *Do you have any emotional problems?* No *How do you respond to stressful circumstances in your life?* Pretty well. *Have you ever been told that you had claustrophobia?* No | Psychiatric history SCUBA diving involves lot of stress and it is essential that the patient is able to cope up with the stress. Underwater panic stress reactions and hyperventilation is most likely to occur in patients who are mentally unfit. |
| *Have you ever been hospitalized overnight?* No *When did you have your last chest-X-ray?* About a year ago. *What was the result?* I was told that it was normal. | PAMP HUGS FOSSED, H for Hospitalizations Avoid body movements that display boredom: wandering eyes around, gazing away from the patient, fiddling with stethoscope, tuning fork, pens etc, stretching, picking at finger nails |

| | |
|---|---|
| *Are you experiencing pain while urinating?*<br>No | U for Urinary symptoms |
| *Have you been nauseated?*<br>No<br>*Have you been vomiting?*<br>No<br>*Are you opening your bowels regularly?*<br>Yes, doctor. | G for Gastrointestinal problems |
| *Have your sleeping patterns changed anyway?*<br>No | S for Sleep problems |
| *What are the main medical problems in your family?*<br>cancer<br>*What type of cancer?*<br>I don't know | F for family history |
| *Are you sexually active?*<br>Yes, with my girl friend<br><br>*Have you ever been diagnosed with an STD?*<br>No | FOSSED: S for Sexual history |
| *Do you smoke?*<br>Yes<br>*How many packs do you smoke per day and for how many years?*<br>One pack per day for the last 8 years.<br><br>*What do you do for a living?*<br>I am an architect.<br><br>*Do you use any recreational drugs?*<br>No<br>*Do you drink alcoholic beverages?*<br>No | Smoking<br>Patients who smoke heavily are probably physically unfit for scuba diving.<br><br><br>Occupation<br><br><br>Drugs<br><br>Alcohol |

| | |
|---|---|
| *Are you involved in any type of exercise?* Yes, I use treadmill for an hour every morning *Have you ever passed out during or after exercise?* No *Have you ever gotten unexpectedly short of breath during or after exercise?* No | Exercise If the applicant is able to swim several laps in the pool without difficulty or jog a mile without collapsing or perform aerobic exercise regularly, he is probably physically fit for scuba diving. Any significant, exercise-limiting problem like angina, heart failure, seizures, pulmonary insufficiency should prohibit scuba diving. |
| *What do you usually eat?* I eat mostly sandwiches, rich with chicken nuggets, bread and butter, and occasionally spaghetti with noodles. *Have you ever developed allergy to any food?* No | FOSSED, D for Diet Exploring dietary habits of the patient helps in recommending dietary changes. (e.g. salt restriction in hypertension, sugar restriction in diabetes, saturated fats restriction in obesity, increasing fiber intake in constipation etc) |
| *You are all excited about SCUBA diving?* Yes, doctor *I can see that, now I will do a physical examination. I will perform all necessary tasks asked for on your medical checkup form. Let me wash my hands.* | Perform all things required to be filled by the physician on the form |
| *Please sit on the end of the table up here* Ok, doctor Perform a physical examination on the patient doing all things asked for on the form. | Only after finishing doing the things asked for on the examination form, should you think about performing other things. Remember time just flies away in the patient encounter. Therefore, doing unasked things first rather than the things asked for on the examination form is simply flirting with disaster. |
| *Now, Mr. Bell, based on the information you have given me and the physical examination I have done, you are physically and mentally fit to undergo* | At the end of the interview, give the patient an opportunity to ask questions |

| | |
|---|---|
| *SCUBA diving training. Do you have any questions for me?* | |
| No doctor, thank you. *Congratulations, all the best, bye-bye.* | Close your encounter with a pleasant smile added with a thank you and a good bye |

# EIGHTH PATIENT ENCOUNTER

Mrs. Roselyn McPherson, mother of a 5-year-old child, John McPherson, came to your clinic to talk about her son's diarrhea. Obtain a focused history from mother, Child not available for physical examination. Discuss your initial diagnostic impression and your workup plan with the mother. After leaving the room, complete your patient note on the form provided.

| | |
|---|---|
| *Hello, Good morning, Mrs. McPherson, I am Dr. Paul. How are you today?*<br>I am fine, thank you, doctor | For all pediatric cases, use the same formula we used for adult cases:<br>**CPR LIQOR FAAA TRIFT PAMP HUGS FOSSED**<br>Under Past medical history, ask BIG FUN<br>Where<br>B—Birth history: Antenatal, Natal, Neonatal<br>I-Immunizations and illnesses<br>G-Growth and development<br>F—Feeding history<br>U—Usual care<br>N—Normal activities |
| *What made you come in today, Mrs. McPherson?*<br>I work 6 days a week, 14 hours a day and we have two other kids beside this baby. My wife has to take them to school and look after them. We take our kids to Nason hospital whenever we get problems and this time we came to this hospital because we heard nice things about this place. We don't know, I am tired to go around the hospitals, this baby has been pooping for a while | Chief complaint<br><br>Dealing with Rambling Patient<br>This parent rambles on and on talking more about his life and his family rather his son's problem. The physician permits this lengthy response because it gives valuable information about the patient's background and parents. |
| *How old is baby John?*<br><br>3 years old | Call the baby with the their name<br>Diarrhea is common, especially during the first 4 years of life. |

| | |
|---|---|
| *When did his diarrhea start?* <br> Two days ago <br> *How did it start, suddenly or gradually?* <br> Suddenly | CPR: P for Present Illness, history of <br> Most cases of diarrhea last 2 to 4 days <br> and are due to a viral cause. <br> Diarrhea may be acute or short term, <br> which is usually related to bacterial or viral <br> infections, or chronic or long-term, which <br> is usually related to functional disorders. |
| *How many stools did he have in the last 24 hours?* <br> about 6 times <br><br> *What is the color of the stools?* <br> Light brown | Indicators of severe diarrhea in children <br> of different ages: <br> In children aged under 1 year, stools >9 <br> in 24 hours <br> In children aged 1-2 years, stools>14 <br> in 24 hours <br> In children aged >2 years, stools>19 in <br> 24 hours |
| *Is it getting better, worse or staying the same?* <br> I think it is getting worse, doctor, because he is very weak and irritable. Also, his mouth is dry and sticky, doctor. I don't know what to do with this. I have two other children who make me busy through the day <br> *Dr: I have young children too, I know what you mean. Now, let me ask few more questions about his diarrhea. Are there pieces of undigested food in the diarrhea?* <br> No, doctor <br> *Have you noticed any blood or pus in the stool?* <br> No <br> *Does he have foul-smelling or oily-looking stools?* <br> No <br> *How were John's bowel habits before diarrhea?* <br> Just normal <br> *Does he have alternating diarrhea and constipation?* <br> No | Listen for any signs of dehydration in mother's descriptions. <br><br><br> Discussing common things without revealing too much personal information is a good way to improve rapport and connection with the patient. <br><br> Children get diarrhea because they don't chew long enough or they drink too much fruit juice and cannot adequately digest their food. <br><br> Malabsorption or celiac disease <br><br> If the child has fewer than one bowel movement every 3 or 4 days and has hard bowel movements, he or she may be constipated. Sometimes, diarrhea follows a period of constipation. |

| | |
|---|---|
| *How many bowel movements did he use to have per day?*<br>2 or 3 | |
| *Now, let us talk about any other problems he has been having lately.*<br>*Has he been vomiting?*<br>No<br>*Does he have cold?*<br>No<br>*Does he have any neck stiffness?*<br>No<br>*Is he also belching and having gas?*<br>No<br>*Does he complain abdominal pain?*<br>No<br>*Does he complain itching in his anal area?*<br>No | Review of Systems<br>The purpose of ROS is to uncover problems that the patient has not brought up, either because she has forgotten the data or considered the data unimportant or irrelevant to the presenting problem. Respiratory infections can present with diarrhea.<br>Intestinal parasites may cause perianal itching and diarrhea. |
| *Did he sustain any injuries or falls?*<br>No | TRIFT: T for Trauma |
| *Good, has he ever developed a rash during the course of this illness?*<br>No | Rash<br>Conditions like anaphylaxis, peanut allergy, fluke infections, helminth infections, kawasaki disease present with diarrhea and rash |
| *Did he drink water from an unfamiliar water source?*<br>As far as I know I can't think of any such possibility.<br>*Is your child in day care or preschool?*<br>We are home schooling him.<br>*Was he exposed to any pets or animals recently?*<br>No | Infections<br><br>Evaluate the possibility of contracting infection from another child in settings like day care centers or preschools because outbreaks or infectious diarrhea are common among children attending childcare centers. |

| | |
|---|---|
| *Has he been running a fever?*<br>I am not sure doctor, but certainly he has been feeling hotter than usual. | F for Fever<br>Rotavirus causes fever in 50% of cases, Escherichia coli in 20% of cases, and Campylobacter in 80% of cases. |
| *Has your family recently returned from a camping trip or foreign travel?*<br>No | T for Travel<br>Traveling to a foreign country or a camping might present with Traveler's diarrhea or Giardiasis |
| *Now, let us talk about his previous medical problems. How has his health been in the past?*<br>He had a diarrhea when he was one and a half-year old baby. It stayed for 3 days and went off by itself.<br>*Does your child have any other disease or illness?*<br>No<br>*Was he ever operated on, even as an infant?*<br>No | PAMP HUGS FOSSED, P for Past Medical History |
| *Was he born at term, or preterm or postterm?*<br>*Term*<br><br>*Were there any problems after the birth like convulsions, jaundice, cyanosis, or feeding difficulties?*<br>No<br><br>*Have the baby had any congenital anomalies?*<br>No | In the past medical history, ask BIG FUN in all pediatric cases.<br>Birth history—antenatal, natal, and neonatal |
| *Is he up to date on his immunizations?*<br>Yes<br>*Did the child develop any reactions to the immunizations?*<br>No | BIGFUN: I for Immunizations |

| | |
|---|---|
| *Is he reaching all milestones on time?*<br>Yes<br><br>*When did he start walking?*<br>At 12 months with one hand held<br><br>*Is he toilet-trained?*<br>He is still learning to use the toilet. | G for Growth and development<br>Encopresis—loss of control of bowel movements—is not uncommon in recently toilet-trained children.<br><br>Most children can control their bowels and are toilet trained by the time they are four years of age. |
| *How is his appetite?*<br>Good<br>*Are you giving any vitamin supplements to the child?*<br>No<br>*Does the diarrhea occur after eating a particular food?*<br>No<br>*Does John drink a lot of juice, sweet drinks and water?*<br>Yes, doctor, most of the time he thrives on juices and sweet drinks.<br>*Has he eaten any sea foods or undercooked hamburger etc?*<br>No | F for Feeding history<br>Food intolerances may cause diarrhea<br><br>Consumption of large amounts of juices or sweet drinks or caffeinated beverages may result in loose stools. |
| *Is he under the regular care of a pediatrician?*<br>Yes<br>*Are you keeping sharp and electrical objects away from your kid?*<br>Yes<br>*Is he protected from heaters, stoves, and other hot objects?*<br>Yes<br>*Are you taking the growth and weight charts for the child?*<br>Yes, they are normal | U for Usual care<br>Make sure the child is proteced well in the home and in the daycare from harmful objects and surfaces. If not, educate the parent. |

| | |
|---|---|
| *Now, about his normal activities. Is the child playful and active or cranky and irritable?*<br>He plays a lot<br><br>*Does the child intermingle with other kids of his age?*<br>Yes | N for Normal activities and behavior |
| *Does he have any allergies, such as to medications, foods, pets, or plants?*<br>No | After BIGFUN, return to PAMP HUGS FOSSED, A for Allergies<br>Allergies may cause diarrhea. Food allergies like lactose intolerance may present with diarrhea. |
| *Is he taking any medications for any kind of problems?*<br>No<br>*Did you give him any medication for this diarrhea?*<br>I've tried some imodium but it did not help him | M for Medications<br>Medications such as amoxicillin, laxatives, stool softeners, mineral oil can cause diarrhea.<br>Besides, knowing what medications the patient already used will spare the embarrasment of prescribing medications the patient has already used prior to coming to the clinic. |
| *Could your child be feeling nervous or anxious for some reason?*<br>Not as I know of him<br>*Does John's diarrhea occur around the time of events that might produce stress, such as school, sports, or performances or travel?*<br>I've not noticed anything of that sort. | PAMP HUGS FOSSED: P for Psych Hx<br>Anxiety, nervousness or excitement that happens on the first day of school can cause problems like diarrhea. |
| *Has he ever been hospitalized for any illnesses or operations?*<br>No | PAMP HUGS FOSSED: H for Hospitalizations |
| *Is the child able to control his bladder?*<br>Yes | |

| | |
|---|---|
| *Does your child have pain below the waist?*<br>No<br>*Does he complain of pain when urinating?*<br>No<br>*Is he urinating more frequently than usual?*<br>No, actually he is urinating less frequently, less than 6 times per day<br>*Is the urine discolored?*<br>No<br>*Does he have bed-wetting?*<br>No | U for Urologic symptoms |
| *Does he have any other belly problems beside diarrhea, like belly pain?*<br>No | G for Gastrointestinal symptoms |
| *How is his sleep?*<br>Good | S for Sleeping patterns<br>Disturbances in sleep could be clues to intestinal worm infections, night terrors etc |
| *Do others in your household have similar symptoms?*<br>No<br>*Do you have other children beside John?*<br>Yes, I have a seven-year old daughter from my previous marriage. | FOSSED: F for Family History<br>The presence of similar illness in other members of the family should prompt you to the possibility of presence of a common source of infection. |
| *Is she healthy?*<br>She is living with her father and I don't want to talk about her. | Don't probe into issues the patient is not comfortable to discuss |
| *Are his genital organs consistent with sexuality?*<br>Yes | S for Sexual history |
| *Is there any exposure to smoking?*<br>I smoke outside the home | S for Social history |

| | |
|---|---|
| | Nicotine can cause diarrhea in young children. Mother's smoking is also related to many health problems in the children. |
| *O.K Mrs. McPherson, you told me that your son John has been suffering from diarrhea for the last 2 days. Most of the diarrheas that affect children of this age groups are due to viral infections. They go away by themselves without any medications. I remember that you told me that he drinks lots of juice and sweet drinks. Right? It may be a cause of his diarrhea.* | Counseling<br>Explain your impression of the child's illness to the parent. |
| *At this time, the most important thing you should do is to make sure that John drinks enough water or other fluids to prevent dehydration. Am I clear? Because that is very important. For rehydration, use only commercially available electrolyte solutions. Don't use sports drinks: their sugar content can make the diarrhea worse.* | The mother or the standardized patient has covertly told you the signs of dehydration in the baby. Therefore, it is vitally important to advice the mother about need for immediate rehydration of the baby. |
| *Soft drinks, juices, soups, sports drinks, and boiled skim milk may make the child sicker. If he doesn't ask for something to drink regularly, give him sips of oral rehydration solution every 10 to 15 minutes. One more thing, do not give him any over-the-counter antidiarrheal drugs.* | Explain the responsibility of the parent while you wait for further action.<br><br>Educate the parent about how to rehydrate her child on a practical basis. |
| *I need to do a physical examination on John. We need to take his blood and stool samples to identify any possible bacterium or parasite responsible for his diarrhea. Before I go, do you have any questions for me?* | Explain the need to perform a physical examination on the child |
| No, thank you, doctor | Ask whether the patient had any questions for you |
| *Thank you, Mrs. McPherson, you have a good evening, bye-bye* | Without abruptly bringing the encounter to an end, say good-bye and a greeting at the end of the interview. |

# NINTH PATIENT ENCOUNTER

Desiree Smith, a 21 year-old female, comes to your clinic complaining of vaginal discharge

Blood pressure = 122/70 Heart Rate = 73 Respirations = 14 Temperature = 98.6

Perform a focused history and physical examination on this patient. After leaving the room, complete your patient note on the form provided.

| | |
|---|---|
| *Good Morning, Ms. Smith, I am Dr. Paul. I will be the physician to take care of you this morning. I am glad to see you this morning.*<br>Thank you, doctor. | Knock on the door before entering the patient examination room, greet and shake the hand of the patient after entering the room. Relax and sit near the patient.<br>Try to sit at the same level as the patient, this helps establish good eye contact during the interview |
| *What is bothering you this morning, Ms.Smith?*<br>I went to grocery store yesterday evening and I developed some itchiness around my vagina. That's not all it is. I had some discharge and it is bothering me a lot, I mean it's like hell. | CPR: C for Chief Complaint<br>Focus your history on the nature of discharge, associated symptoms, sexual history and other medical conditions. Vaginitis is the most common women's health problem. So, well prepare for this case in Step-2 CS.<br>'Hell' is a common word in the pain vocabulary of the patients in the United States. It describes the intensity of patient's suffering.<br>What to ask for in a patient with discharge? An easy mnemonic would be, DISCHARGE |
| *Since how long have you had this discharge?*<br>For the last 10 days.<br>*Is the problem getting better, worse, or staying the same?*<br>It seems to be getting worse<br>*You told me about itching. Can you describe a bit?* | **D for Duration** |

My vagina is very itchy, particularly on the outer fold of the vagina it is more bothersome. I got some kind of vaginal discharge six months ago. I went to a doctor in Pennsylvania. He prescribed a drug, which cured me of that discharge.

*What is the smell of the discharge?*
Oh, for the last 10 days I have had fishy smell from my vaginal area.

*What is the color of the discharge?*
First it was white, then yellow and now I have been having a greenish-yellow discharge, thin and creamy.

*Do you have fever?*
I don't know, but I feel warm

*Is it light or heavy?*
It's heavy, an also I did notice that 'air bubbles' were coming from my vagina.

*Have you ever developed a rash during the course of this illness?*
I am not sure, the skin on the outside of my vagina has started to flake a little. I have also noticed what seems to be a rash, many small red dots, and this is dotted around the outside of my vagina, particularly in the area between my vagina and anus.

*Do you have any ulcers over the vulva or the area around the vagina?*
No, doctor.

**I for Itching**
Patients with vaginal infections usually present with intense vulvar itching.

**S for Smell**
Bacterial vaginosis—fishy or musty odor
Candidal vaginosis—Usually no smell.
Trochomonas vaginalis—malodorous

**C for Color and Consistency**
Discharge of Trichomonas vaginalis ranges in color from white to yellow, gray, or green and is frothy and sticky.
Discharge of Bacterial Vaginosis is usually thin, white-yellow or gray, homogeneous, and moderately increased in volume over the patient's normal discharge.
Discharge of Candidal vaginitis is usually thick, white and curdy like cotton cheese.
Discharge of chlamydial cervicitis is mucopurulent.
Foreign body (lost tampon) causes a foul-smelling black discharge

**H for Heat (Fever)**
Conditions like PID, toxic shock syndrome, infected IUD present with vaginal discharge and fever

**A for Amount**
A certain amount of vaginal discharge is normal, increased amounts should raise the suspicion of infection or other more serious disorders
Suspect Trichomoniasis in patient complaining of profuse, bubbly, frothy white discharge

**R for Rash**
Illnesses like Syphilis, Toxic shock syndrome present may present with a rash.

*How is this affecting your daily life?*
I am very frustrated, doctor. I have become so exasperated with this, it really bothers me so much.
*I understand, Ms.Smith it is a truly frustrating problem. Do not worry, let us work together to bring out best possible outcome. OK , now*

**G for Genital Ulcers**
Herpes simplex types 1 and 2 may cause genital ulceration.
Vulvar ulcerations can be seen in all stages of syphilis.
**E for Effect on daily life**
Sympathize with the patient whenever they express their exasperation.

*Do you have any other complaints?*
I have vaginal burning and pain around the vagina. Also, I have lots of lower back pain. I also feel dizzy.

*What do you mean by dizzy?*
I become physically exhausted after some work.

*Do you have any skin infections?*
No
*Do you have any joint pains?*
No

R for Review of Systems
Common words mean different things to different people. Ask the patient the meaning of their words. e.g. dizziness means lightheadedness for some, exhaustion for others
'gas' means abdominal bloating for some, farting for others
'constipation' means no bowel movement for 2 days for some, as many as 7 days for others

Skin infections can alter the barrier function of skin through persistent moisture and development of maceration, and predispose to vaginal infections.
Disseminated gonorrhea may present with skin lesions and joints pains: Arthritis-dermatitis syndrome.

*Now, let me ask you a few questions about your past health.*
*Do you have any other diseases you can think of beside this illness?*

PAMP HUGS FOSSED: Past Medical Hx
Don't grill the patient with all kinds of questions to obtain unwanted information. Remember there is not much time left.

| | |
|---|---|
| No | Patients with recurrent vaginal infections should be evaluated for diabetes mellitus. |
| *Have you ever been tested for HIV?*<br>No<br>*Did you ever have vaginal disease before?*<br>Yes, 6 months ago I was treated for some yeast infection in the vagina. | Diabetes mellitus, immunosuppressive disorders, anemias, HIV can act as predisposing factors to vaginal infections |
| *Did you receive any treatment for that illness?*<br>It really went wild at that time, I was losing concentration on things I do, I was getting tired so quickly after I start doing something. I finally went to a doctor and she put me on Diflucan 100 mg one a day for three weeks.<br>*Did it clear up?*<br>Yes | Give the patient time to explain their answers to your questions. Wait and maintain silence for sometime to help the patient express herself. |
| *Do you have any allergies, such as to medications, foods, pets, or plants?*<br>Yes, Aspirin<br><br>*What happens when you take aspirin?*<br>I get stomach discomfort | A for Allergies<br>Most patients interpret side-effects of medications as allergies. Therefore, it is important to ask what exactly happens when the patient takes the medication. Often, patient had a side-effect to the medication, not allergy |
| *Are you taking any medications for this problem?*<br>I got a vaginal spray from Rite Aid, but it hasn't seemed to help. | M for Medications<br>Many women try over-the-counter products to treat vaginitis. |
| *Are you on oral contraceptives?*<br>No | Oral contraceptive use is a predisposing factor to vaginal infections. |
| *Have you been feeling depressed lately?*<br>Not really but certainly I lost interest in some activities because of the discharge. | P for Psychological symptoms<br>It is not unusual that many patients with gynecological disorders, especially with |

| | chronic ailments, feel depressed about their situation. |
|---|---|
| *Have you ever been hospitalized overnight?*<br>No | H for Hospitalizations |
| *Have you noticed any change in the frequency of urination after this illness?*<br>Yes, I am feeling as if I need to urinate more often than usual.<br>*Are you experiencing pain while urinating?*<br>No<br>*Have you noticed any change of color of urine?*<br>No | U for Urological symptoms<br>Symptoms of urethral irritation—dysuria, frequency, and urgency are additional symptoms of vaginosis. |
| *Did you feel sick to your stomach?*<br>sometimes<br><br>*Are you opening your bowels regularly?*<br>Yes | G for Gastrointestinal symptoms<br>PID may present with vaginal discharge and abdominal pain<br>It is also important to ask for gastrointestinal symptoms because patients who involve in oral-genital sexual activity may present GI symptoms along with genital discharge e.g. Gonorrhea. |
| *How is your sleep?*<br>I can't sleep well due to irritation down there | S for Sleeping pattern |
| *Does anyone among your family have this or a similar problem?*<br>I am staying in our college dorm now away from my family. I do not know whether any of them have the same problem.<br>*Are there any illnesses that run in your family?*<br>No | FOSSED: F for Family History |

| | |
|---|---|
| *Now, I would like to ask you a few questions about your reproductive health. When was your most recent menstrual period?*<br>2 weeks ago<br>*Are your cycles regular?*<br>Yes<br>*How many days are in your cycle?*<br>29 days<br>*Is the bleeding heavy or light?*<br>light<br>*Any pain with bleeding?*<br>No<br>*Do you use tampons?*<br>No | O for Ob/Gyn Hx<br><br><br><br><br><br><br><br><br><br><br>Chemicals and objects like tampons, toilet tissue, contraceptives, or other objects left in the vagina longer than necessary may cause irritations that lead to vaginitis. |
| *Have you noticed any relation between your vaginal discharge and menstruation?*<br>Not really, doctor.<br>*Have you ever been pregnant?*<br>No<br>*When was your last pap smear?*<br>Two months ago<br>*Normal or abnormal?*<br>Normal | Pelvic inflammatory disease usually begins shortly after a menstrual period. Recurrences of Herpes simplex are correlated with stress and the premenstrual cycle.<br><br>Ask all women about their last Pap smear, if they are not getting it, recommend it. |
| *Do you smoke?*<br>No<br><br>*What do you do for a living?*<br>I am a college student. But, I work part-time in a t-shirt making shop<br><br>*Does this problem interfere with your job?*<br>Yes, doctor, I am not able to concentrate on my job or studies. I must get rid of this bad stuff in my body immediately. | S for Social History—SODA<br>S for Smoking<br><br><br>O for Occupation |

| | |
|---|---|
| *Do you use any illegal drugs?* <br> No | D for Drugs |
| *Do you drink alcohol?* <br> No | A for Alcohol |
| *Now, I would like to ask you a few questions regarding your sexual life. I know that is a sensitive, private issue. But it will help me get a total picture of your health. So, is it all right with you?* <br> Yes, doctor. <br><br> *You told me a while ago that you have been sexually active. Right? Does your sexual activities involve vaginal intercourse?* <br> Yes <br><br> *How many sex partners you have?* <br> Just one <br><br> *Do you use any sex toys?* <br> Never <br><br> *Have you been sexually active during the last six months?* <br> Yes, but I tried having sex once and it was painful. <br><br> *Has your sexual partner been tested to ensure that you are not becoming reinfected?* <br> No | PAMP HUGS FOSSED: S for Sexual Hx <br> Use a transitive as you move from one area to the other <br><br> Explore patient's sexual practices, number of partners, using protective barriers etc <br><br> Sexually transmitted infections like Trichomoniasis are known to spread by exchanging fluids through vaginal intercourse, sharing sex toys and mutual masturbation. <br><br> Dyspareunia is common in vaginal infections <br><br> Yeast infections usually aren't caught from a sex partner but Trichomonas vaginalis is transmitted through coitus. <br><br> Testing and treatment of sex partners is essential in infections like Trichomoniasis to prevent reinfection |
| *Are you involved in any type of physical activity like exercise?* <br> I used to run a mile every morning before getting this illness. | E for Exercise |

| | |
|---|---|
| *Have you changed your eating habits any way?*<br>No<br><br>*Tell me something about your diet?*<br>I just eat regular foods, but I've started to eat organic foods recently | D for Diet<br>Exploring dietary habits of the patient helps in recommending dietary changes. (e.g. salt restriction in hypertension, sugar restriction in diabetes, saturated fats restriction in obesity, increasing fiber intake in constipation etc) |
| *Now I want to do a physical examination on you. After that I will tell you about my impressions of your condition and what I am going to do from that point. OK?, let me wash my hands . . . .*<br>Perform abdominal examination<br>Listen to heart and lungs<br>*"Let me untie your gown so that I can listen to your lungs"*<br>Ok<br>*"Can you move your breast so that I can listen to your heart?"*<br>No problem, Doc<br>*"Later I will also perform the examination of your genitals to see the effect of the disease. Alright?"*<br>Ok | WPSCF: W for Washing hands, and P for<br>Physical examination<br>Let the patient know what you are going to do from point to point.<br><br>Try to be communicative during the physical examination. You do not have to ask for permission for every little thing you do.<br><br>Do not make an attempt to make all possible observations but only those that are relevant to the problems at hand.<br><br>Do not try to perform pelvic examination. But tell the patient that you are needed to perform it in order to evaluate her condition. |
| *So, Ms. Smith, let me summarize your problems briefly. You told me that you have vaginal discharge for the last 10 days which is getting worse, it has, fishy smell with greenish yellow color and air bubbles, you also have vaginal burning and low back pain. Right?*<br>Yes | S: S for Summary |
| *Well, Ms.Smith, thank you for your cooperation during the history taking and physical examination. Based upon the information you have given me and* | Closing the encounter:<br>1. Thank the patient for the cooperation |

*the examination I have done, I have some possibilities in my mind. One is you can be having Bacterial vaginosis, which is caused by several bacteria and the other being trichomoniasis which is a disease that usually spread by sexual contact. I also need to perform a vaginal inspection and examination to get the comprehensive idea of your illness. In addition, I would like to do some tests to confirm the diagnosis. Depending on our final diagnosis of your condition it might be necessary that both you and your partner get treatment, because you may become infected again if your partner isn't treated. Am I clear?*

Yes

*Do you have any questions or concerns for me?*

Yes, doctor, what can I do to prevent the re-infections?

*That is a very good question, Ms. Smith, you should take proper hygiene of the vaginal area because improper hygiene and uncleanness are the main factors in the causation of re-infection. Wipe from front to back when bathing and after urination and defecation. Wear cotton underpants. Because infectious agents develop more quickly in moisture, keep the area around the genitals as dry as possible. Do not start your sexual activities until you get rid of this infection and also always use protective measures when engaging in sexual contact. For example encourage your partner to wear a condom during the intercourse. And as I mentioned earlier, if we find trich in you, we should treat your partner. Am I clear?*

Yes doctor, thank you

*See you later, Good bye*

2. In addition, use terms like 'we', 'our', 'us' to connote to the patient that both of you are working together for the benefit of the patient.
3. Answer patient questions
4. Close the interview with a pleasant thank you and goodbye

Answer every question immediately. Appreciate the patient for asking the question.
Explain your answer using simple terminology.

Wearing of occlusive clothing made of synthetic materials may cause atrophic vaginitis.

WPSCF: F for Farewell

# TENTH PATIENT ENCOUNTER

Mrs. Martha Gabriel, a 65 year-old female, comes to your office complaining of headache. She is new to your practice.

Blood pressure=134/83 Heart Rate = 89 Respirations = 15 Temperature = 98.7

Perform a focused history and physical examination on this patient. After leaving the room, complete your patient note on the form provided.

| | |
|---|---|
| *Hello, Good Morning, Mrs. Gabriel, I am Dr. Paul, glad to see you this morning.* Thank you, doctor | Using their last name—not first name unless they give permission to do so—introduce yourself to the patient. |
| *So, what brings you here today, Mrs. Gabriel?* Doctor, I feel so tired. | In every patient, start with CPR Chief Complaint All symptoms should be explored to avoid ambiguity and vagueness. Patients use vague words to describe their problems. For example, tiredness has different meanings: lack of interest in work, feeling bored, shortness of breath with exertion, feeling tired after some walk, headache etc. |
| *Dr: Can you tell me more about your tiredness?* Pt: Yes, I am tired of these headaches | Explore what the patient exactly mean by their words. Prevalence of migraines is 2-3 times higher in women. Migraine occurs mainly in women Cluster headaches occur mainly in men |
| *When did it start?* This morning *Usually, how long does each attack of headache last?* Around 3 to 6 hours | Take history carefully because history by far provides the most useful information for evaluating a headache. Cluster headaches last 30-90 minutes while migraine headaches 4-24 hours Migraine headaches may begin at any age between the ages of five and 35. |

*Since how long have you been having headaches?*
For the last 35 years.

*Are they getting better, worse, or staying the same?*
They are getting worse

*Have you been evaluated before for those headaches?*
No

*Have there been intervals of weeks or months without the headache?*
No, they come almost every week.

*How old were you when you got these kind of headaches for the first time in your life?*
The first headaches started when I was 34 years old, and I remember because I had virtually never had a headache before then, so it was surprising.

*Do you have sensitivity to light?*

Yes

*Is there any warning of the attack?*
Yes, doctor, before the headache starts, sometimes I become sensitive to light, I see blurriness, dazzling zigzag lines, and blind spots before my eyes. And, I forgot to tell you, it is slightly painful when I touch my head with my hands.

*Are you aware of any factors that can bring on these headaches?*
No

Blurring of vision is frequent in Migraine headaches while infrequent in cluster headaches.

Ask for any prodromal warning of some kind, which precede the headache.

Scalp tenderness is common in migraine.

Withdrawal from alcohol, caffeine, drugs, tobacco may bring on headaches.

Explore the impact of the illness on the patient's life to estimate the severity of the disease

| | |
|---|---|
| *What do these headaches keep you from doing?*<br>Almost everything, doc. I throw up and go to bed. That's it for the day. I can't even help my daughter doing her homework. It is that bad | |
| *Can you think of any other problems you've had recently?*<br><br>*Do you have any confusion?*<br>Yes<br>*Do you have any weakness of an arm or leg?*<br>Yes<br>*Do you have tingling of face or hands?*<br>Yes<br>*Do you have any nasal congestion?*<br>No | CPR: R for Review of Systems<br>Classic migraine is characterized by the appearance of an 'aura' 10-30 minutes before the classic migraine attack. Patient may see zigzag lines, flashing lights in front of his eyes. Other symptoms include confusion, speech difficulty, tingling of face or hands, and weakness of an arm or leg.<br>Nasal congestion and eye watering are more common in cluster headaches than migraine headaches.<br>Exertion due to cough and sneezing can induce acute exertional headache. |
| *Now let me ask you more direct questions about your headache. Where is your headache located?*<br>On the right side of my head.<br><br>*Do they come on your right side every time you get a headache?*<br>No, some time on the left, but most often on the right side. | Now, ask for LIQOR FAAA TRIFT<br>L for Location<br>Tension headaches are usually described as a continuous pain or tightness over the entire head<br>Migraine headaches are a severe, throbbing pain over one of both temples.<br>Cluster headaches are always one-sided, around the eyes.<br>Migraine headaches are typically unilateral at the beginning of a single attack, but they often generalize and most patients will have attacks on both sides of the head. |

| | |
|---|---|
| *If 10 is the worst pain you've ever had, where is the pain of this headache on a scale of 1 to 10?* probably 8 | I for Intensity Asking for the intensity of the pain helps determine the severity of headache. |
| *What kind of pain are you experiencing with the headache? Can you describe it a bit?* It is difficult to find words, doctor, its kind a throbbing headache pounding around my forehead. I can feel my head vessels pulsating with pain. I feel somebody stabbing on my head with a knife. | Quality When patient describes a throbbing, pounding headache with pulsating vessels over the scalp, think of migraine |
| *How does your headache begin—suddenly or slowly?* Sometimes suddenly and sometimes slowly.<br><br>*When does the headache occur?* Most of the times they start when I wake up from my sleep, sometimes they also occur later in the day when I return to my home from my work. | O for Onset Migraine often starts on waking up in the morning, but can occur later in the day. |
| *Does the headache seem to spread and travel to other areas during the course of attack? or does it stay in one place?*<br><br>Yes, doctor, it started on one side and moved to the other. Sometimes, the pain goes from my temples on each side to behind my ears. | R for Radiation A migraine typically begins in a specific area on one side of the head, then spreads to the other side, builds in intensity over 1 to 2 hours and then gradually subsides. |
| *How often do you get these headaches?* I had three real bad ones within two weeks time. I threw up with them and had to go to bed with them. | F for Frequency<br><br>Cluster headaches occur 1-6 times per day for several weeks. Migraine headaches occur 1-10 timer per month. |

| | |
|---|---|
| *Do you have them every week, or every month or every couple of months?*<br>I get the damn thing all the time, almost every week | |
| *Does anything make your headache worse?*<br>Yes, doctor, if I put my head down, or stand up too fast, it feels as though my head is filled with water, extremely heavy. | A for Aggravating factors<br>Standing up, bending, straining, coughing, sneezing, lifting, running may aggravate headaches.<br>Bright lights, noise, and alcohol can trigger a migraine.<br>Moving around can make the migraine headache feel worse |
| *Have you learnt or developed any special techniques to get some relief from these headaches?*<br>Yes, I lie down in my bedroom with lights off and putting a cold compress on my forehead. Sometimes, when that does not work, I am massaging my head with a lot of pressure. I am sleeping in the process, and when I get up, my headache is gone. | A for Alleviating factors<br>Usually, patient with cluster headache paces and pounds their fist, while patient with migraine rests in a quiet, dark room.<br><br>Sleeping, lying down in a dark, quiet room, putting a cold compress over the forehead, massaging the scalp alleviate the pain of migraine. |
| *Do you have any other complaints that you think associated with your headaches?*<br><br>Doctor, I am sensitive to light and noise. Sometimes, I feel I had no calories in my body. My hands and feet are becoming cold and sweaty.<br><br>*Do you get any problems with your eyes when you get a headache?*<br>Yes, doctor, there have been times when my left eye would hurt, or my vision would be blurry. Light bothers me a lot | A for Association factors<br><br>Migraine headaches are often accompanied by nausea and vomiting. Also phonophobia and photophobia are commonly associated with migraine. |

| | |
|---|---|
| *What happens with the light?*<br>It's like a glare, I can't stand it. | |
| *Have you ever had a head injury or concussion?*<br>No | TRIFT: T for Trauma<br>History of trauma is very important to ask for in all patients who complain of headaches because headaches are the most frequent and most troubling manifestations of head trauma as part of postconcuccive syndrome. |
| *Have you ever developed a rash during your headaches?*<br>No | R for Rash<br>Headache and rash may be the initial manifestations of some infections like meningitis, e.g. meningococcal meningitis. |
| *Have you ever had a sinusitis or sinus infection?*<br>No | I for Infections<br>Sinus headaches may mimic migraines. It typically occurs in the area of sinuses-<br>In the area of the cheeks: Maxillary sinus<br>Bridge of the nose: Ethmoid sinus<br>Above the eyes: Frontal sinus<br>Behind the eyes: Sphenoid sinus |
| *Have you been running a fever in addition to your headache?*<br>No, doctor | F for Fever<br>Ask about fever in every patient with headache, because acute febrile illnesses may present with vascular-type throbbing headaches.<br>If the patient has headache, fever, altered mental status, and neck stiffness, suspect *meningitis.* |
| *Did you travel anywhere recently?*<br>I drove to my mom's home last weekend in Miami, Florida.<br><br>*Does your headache affect your driving or travel in any way?*<br>Yes, doctor, between I got the warning signs of nausea and vomiting when I | T for Travel history<br>Since headaches have been associated with travel, vacations, holidays, weekends and other periods of relaxation, the patient should be asked about these associations. |

| | |
|---|---|
| started at my home in Pensacola. Between Ocala and Tampa, I temporarily lost some of my vision, especially my side vision. | Temporary loss of vision, especially side vision, is common in classic migraine. |
| *Now, let me ask about your past illnesses. Do you have any health problems before?*<br>No<br>*Any heart disease or lung disease or hypertension?*<br>No<br>*You never had a stroke?*<br>No | PAMP HUGS FOSSED, P for Past Medical History |
| *Do you have any allergies, such as to medications, foods, pets, or plants?*<br>No | A for Allergies<br>Allergic reactions may present with headaches |
| *Are you taking any medications now?*<br>I have been using analgesics, my daughter bought in Walgreens. But they do not seem to help.<br><br>*Are you using any other medications beside analgesics?*<br>No | M for Medications<br>Self-medication is common in the patients with headache. Failure of analgesics in an emotionally healthy patient with recurring headaches is almost diagnostic of migraine.<br><br>It is important to ask the patient routinely about the drugs when evaluating headache. Nalidixic acid, Oral contraceptives, Cimetidine, Fenfluramine, Nifedipine(Adalat), pain medications, Theophylline, indomethacin, nitroglycerin, reserpine containing medications may act as migraine triggers. Also, if analgesics are overused, they can actually cause headaches. |
| *Describe your mental status before getting a headache? I mean, how do you feel before a headache?*<br>I feel stressful sometimes, but most of the times I feel relaxed. | P for Psychiatric symptoms<br>Stress and time pressure, anger and conflict may act as triggers for causing migraine. |

*Do you experience any hallucinations before you get a headache?*
Yes, doctor, sometimes I see bizarre figures changing shapes and moving across my visual fields.

*Do you fear a dreaded cause such as a tumor in your head responsible for your headaches?*
Yes, doctor, could you please refer me to a neurologist immediately?

*I understand your concerns, Mrs. Gabriel, but there are many reasons for headache. So, first let us decide what exactly is the reason for your headaches. If you need a neurological consultation I certainly refer you one.*

Some patients with migraine may also feel depressed, irritable, and restless.

Fortification hallucinations—slowly enlarging scotomata that are surrounded by luminous angles and that slowly change shape and appear to move across the visual fields—are almost specific for migraine.

Explore the fears of the patient.
It is not uncommon that patients with severe headaches request you for a referral to a neurologist. Acknowledge their concerns and sympathetically advice them what you are going to do if necessary

---

*Have you ever been hospitalized overnight?*
No

H for Hospitalizations
Asking about hospitalizations sometimes help the patient recall other past diseases they forgot to talk about otherwise.

---

*Are you experiencing pain or increased frequency with your urination?*
I do not have pain but sometimes it seems that I am going to bathroom more often than usual.

U for Urinary complaints
During the headache phase of a *common* migraine, the patient may have increased urination. Also, an increase in the frequency or volume of urination is a common warning sign for an impending migraine.

---

*Do you have some nausea?*
Yes, I have nausea and getting a bitter-tasting fluid filling my mouth.

*Do you have vomitings?*
What?

*Are you throwing up?*
No

G for Gastrointestinal complaints
During the headache phase of a *classic* migraine, the patient may have abdominal pain and diarrhea.
85% of patients with migraine also have nausea and vomiting where as only 2-5% of patients with cluster headaches present with those symptoms.

| | Reword your questions whenever the patient do not understand your questions or statements. Primary physicians spend the largest part of their time talking with patients. Therefore, good communication skills are vital for the practice. |
|---|---|
| *Now, let me ask you a few questions about your sleeping habits. Have your sleeping patterns changed in any way?* No | S for Sleep pattern<br>Too much, too little or interrupted sleep can act as a migraine trigger. |
| *Do you have problems falling asleep, staying asleep, or waking up?* No<br><br>*Do you nap in the daytime?* No | Frequent naps during the day may reduce sound sleep at night resulting in a morning headache. An unusual lengthy period of sleep may provoke migraine.<br><br>Cluster headaches frequently occur at night, often at the same time each day, while migraine headaches occur at any time. |
| *Has anyone in your family had history of headaches?* No<br>*In your family, what are the main medical problems?* My dad has high blood pressure and my mum has diabetes | F for Family history<br>Family history of headaches is positive in 90% of patients with migraine and 7% of patients with cluster headaches. |
| *When was your last menstrual period?* 18 years ago.<br><br>*Have you noticed any change in the presentation of your headaches after your menopause?* Little bit, not too much<br><br>*When was your last Pap smear?* Last December | O for Ob/Gyn Hx<br>Menopause due to frank estrogen deficiency is associated with migraine headaches.<br>In premenopausal women, over half of women with migraine report an association between their headaches and their menstrual cycle.<br>Changes in the levels of ovarian hormones and prolactin during pregnancy may modify the course of a migraine. |

136

| | |
|---|---|
| *How was it?* <br> Just normal | Ask about Pap smears in all women |
| *Now, Mrs. Gabriel, I would like to ask you a few questions regarding your sexual life. Is it OK with you?* <br> Yes, doctor. <br><br> *Have you noticed any relation between your sexual activities and your headaches?* <br> No | S for Sexual history <br> Orgasm may produce exertional headaches; withdrawal from sex, also, may produce headaches. <br><br> In younger patients, the frequency and severity of migraine is increased commonly with the use of oral contraceptive pills. |
| *Now, Mrs. Gabriel, let me ask you a few questions about your social life. Do you smoke?* <br> Yes <br> *How many packs?* <br> less than a pack <br><br> *For how many years have you been smoking?* <br> For the last 10 years <br><br> *What sort of work do you do?* <br> I work as a dean of the students in an arts college. <br> *Are you exposed to any stress in your work place?* <br> No, I enjoy my job unless I am sick. <br><br> *How are these headaches currently affecting your job?* <br> Yes, doctor, I can't tell you, doctor, they are showing me the hell I never imagined. I can't stay on the computer as long as I used to, and keeping the deadlines has become a struggle. I am feeling tired and confused, sometimes I am becoming sweaty and even small light or noise is wreaking havoc around me. | Social history—SODA <br><br> S for Smoking <br><br> Smoking can act as a migraine trigger. Many cluster headache patients are heavy smokers and alcohol drinkers. <br><br> O for Occupation <br><br> Stress may act as a trigger or aggravate headaches. <br><br> Severe headaches affect patient's job performance |

| | |
|---|---|
| *Are you exposed to any chemicals or gases at your work place?* (laughter) No, I work inside my air-conditioned office. | Exposure to chemical like nitrites, nitrates, lead, or gases like carbon monoxide may cause headache. A closed room heated by a space heater provides a typical setting for exposure to high levels of carbon monoxide, which triggers headaches. |
| *Do you use any recreational drugs?* No | |
| | D for Drugs Withdrawal of recreational drugs can cause headaches. |
| *Do you drink alcohol?* No, never | |
| | A for Alcohol Alcohol can worsen headaches and provoke them. Typically, alcohol provokes cluster headache. |
| Doctor, I have a question. I am afraid of lung cancer. What is the best method of preventing lung cancer? *That is a very good question, Mrs. Gabriel, more than 80% of lung cancers are related to cigarette smoking, and therefore should be preventable. So, the best method of preventing lung cancer is to stop smoking. Am I clear?* Yes, doctor. | Remember, in Step-2 CS, all patient questions are pre-planned. You must not ignore them lest you suffer penalty. |
| *Do you exercise regularly?* Yes, doctor, I go to gym 3 or 4 times a week. | PAMP HUGS FOSSED—E for Exercise Asking for the possibility of exertional headache. Acute exertional headaches occur with activities such as straining, lifting weights, running, bending, orgasm etc, and they are presumably due to intracranial-spinal pressure dissociations. |
| *Do you experience headaches during exercise with activities like lifting weights etc?* No, doctor | |
| *Have you noticed getting headache after eating specific substances?* Sometimes after eating chocolate or ice cream | D for Diet Explore any relationship between certain foods and headaches. Foods such as alcohol, chocolate, aged cheeses, fermented or marinated foods, |

| | MSG found in Chinese food, artificial sweeteners such as aspartame may trigger migraine headaches. |
| | Also, diary products such as ice cream, milk, yogurt, whipped cream, accent seasoning, Lawry's Seasoned salt may act as migraine triggers. |
| | Hunger, fasting and beverages can act as migraine triggers. |
| *Now, Mrs.Gabriel, let me do a physical on you. Please climb up here and just sit there. Let me wash my hands?*<br>Physical examination in headache includes:<br>*"I am going to look into your eyes with this instrument"*<br>Ophthalmoscopy<br>Fundi for papilloedema, any changes resembling hypertension, any changes suggestive of glaucoma( deep cupping of disc)<br>Pupillary response to light with a flash light<br>Skull for any evidence of trauma<br>Cranial nerves<br>Eyes for refraction problems and visual fields<br>Ears, Nose, Throat, Teeth, Sinuses<br>Cervical movements<br>Neck stiffness<br>Deep tendon reflexes<br>Muscle strength in arms and legs | WPSCF: W for Washing hands, P for Physical examination<br><br>Physical examination is another opportunity to ask history. You can also use that time to do ROS. For example, if you are examining the eyes, it is ok to ask, *'Do you have any problems with your vision now or in the past?'*<br><br>Mouth: teeth may be the source of headache. |
| *So, Mrs. Gabriel, you've told me that you have getting these headaches for the last 35 years, they are getting worse, comes two or three times every week and of 8/10 intensity preceded by sensitivity to light, dazzlingly zig zag lines.* | WPSCF: Summary and Closure<br><br>Summary can be done at any part of the interview where you want to recap the information you obtained with the patient |

*Well, Mrs. Gabriel, based on the information you shared with me and the physical examination I have done I suppose that you are suffering from migraine headaches. You have the characteristic symptoms that are suggestive of migraine headaches. But, before I confirm that diagnosis I need to run a few diagnostic studies to rule out other possibilities. I am going to order a CT scan of your head to rule out any tumors in your head.*

*Please keep a 'headache calendar' which help me find the right treatment for you. Document the time of day, your location (at home, at work, at the bank etc) and your activity when the migraine started. You told me that you eat a lot of chocolate and ice cream. Unfortunately, chocolate and ice cream are found to be the triggers of migraine. I advice you to eliminate or decrease them from your diet. We will meet again when the results of your tests are available. Before I leave, do you have any questions for me?*

No, doctor, thank you.

Always use language the patient can understand. Translate the medical terms that pop up in your mind and describe them in layman language.

*I forgot to tell you. You told me you have been smoking. Would like to stop smoking?*

No, doctor, not now

*Fine, if you change your mind, let me know. We have a wonderful smoking cessation program in our hospital. Thank you, bye, bye*

Some patients do not stop smoking

Good bye, Doc

Close your patient encounter with a pleasant smile added with a thank you and good bye

# TELEPHONE INTERVIEW

A few minutes ago your nurse received a phone call from Mr. Tony Hudson, who is anxious and wants to talk with you as soon as possible. Talk with this patient over the telephone and advise him according to his pertinent history and complaints. You do not need to perform a physical examination for this patient encounter.

| | |
|---|---|
| *Hello*<br>Yes, I am Mr.Tony Hudson, I want to talk to Dr.Paul<br>*Yes, this is Dr.Paul. Good morning, Mr. Tony Hudson.*<br>Good morning, doctor. | Take the telephone and introduce yourself to the patient. Greet him and ask for the presenting complaint. |
| *How can I help you this morning, Mr. Hudson?*<br>Doctor, I am little concerned about my blood pressure. | CPR: Chief complaint<br>After greeting the patient, ask for the chief complaint |
| *Do you have high blood pressure?*<br>Yes, doctor<br>*Since how long?*<br>For the last 5 years.<br><br>*Are you taking any measures to control your blood pressure?*<br>Yes, doctor, I am taking hydrochloro-thiazide 12.5 mg once daily and Inderal 20mg twice a day. | CPR: Present Illness |
| *You told me that you are little concerned about your high blood pressure. What aspect of the high blood pressure is troubling you most?*<br>I am worrying more about the side effects of my blood pressure. I am 44 years old and my life is messy. I damn this dirty life! | When the patient shares his concerns about a particular problem, try to excavate the true source of patient's concerns. |
| *Do not worry, Mr.Hudson, I understand that you are not comfortable with what is going on in your life. Let us work for the better!, Mr.Hudson, what is bothering you most?* | When the patient is low spirited, tell some words of comfort and reassurance. |

I've a sensitive problem. I don't think it is related but I have been concerned about it.

*Go ahead, I am listening.*
I am finding it difficult to maintain my erection.

Most patients with sexual problems feel apprehensive to talk about their problems. The doctor should make the patient ease to discuss freely.

*You are finding it difficult to get the erection or maintain the erection?*
I am able to get the erection but I am not able to maintain it.

Impotence of abrupt onset is usually due to a psychogenic cause where as that of insidious onset is due to an organic cause.

*Did your problem start suddenly or gradually?*
Gradually

Consider impotence when the patient complains consistent inability to maintain an erect penis with sufficient rigidity to allow sexual intercourse.

*Since how long?*
For the last 2 to 3 months

*Is it worsening or staying the same?*
It is worsening.

Episodic or transient impotence is due to a psychogenic cause while persistent impotence with progressive deterioration is due to an organic cause.

*Is your problem occasional or continuos?*
Continuos

*Do you have any pain during intercourse?*
No

*Have you had normal erections before?*
Yes

Never underestimate the importance of history and physical examination, no matter how many technological devices you got in your disposal. About 70% of diagnoses are made on the basis of a proper history and over 90% are made on the bais of history and physical examination.

*How would you describe the quality of your erections in terms of, say, percentage, 40%, 50%, 60% like that?*
May be around 30%

*Once you get an erection how long are you able to maintain it?*
Around 1 minute

Loss of interest in sexual activity is consistent with either psychological etiology or hypogonadism.

| | |
|---|---|
| *Have you noticed any decrease in your interest in sexual activity?*<br>No, doctor | |
| *Have you had any nipple discharge or breast enlargement?*<br>No | CPR: R for Review of Systems<br>Suspect an organic cause of impotence if the patient reports change in the size of his genitals. |
| *Have you noticed any change in the size of your genital organs?*<br>No | Hyperprolactinemia, galactorrhea may present with gynecomastia, nipple discharge and impotence. |
| *Were you involved in any accidents recently or trauma to your back?*<br>Yes, doctor, I was involved in a motorcycle crash two months ago.<br><br>*Did you sustain any injuries?*<br>Yes, doctor, I had an injury to my back.<br><br>*Was your injury evaluated by any health care provider?*<br>No, doctor. I applied some bandage to my back and did not bother to go to a doctor at that time.<br>*Have you noticed any relation between your erectile problems and your accident?*<br>No, doctor | History of trauma<br>Remember to ask for trauma history in all patients presenting with trauma<br>Spinal cord injuries as a result of trauma may result in impotence.<br><br><br>Take notes of important points while maintaining enough eye contact with the patient. |
| *Have you ever had problems with your erection previously?*<br>No, never<br><br>*Do you have any diseases beside your high blood pressure?*<br>No<br><br>*Heart problems, diabetes, nerve disorders, nothing?*<br>Nothing | PAMP HUGS FOSSED, P for Past Medical Hx<br><br>Diabetes mellitus, atherosclerosis and various vasculitides may cause impotence. Neurologic diseases like stroke, multiple sclerosis, sensory nerve damage, anterior temporal lobe lesions may result in impotence. |

| | |
|---|---|
| *Have you ever undergone any operation?*<br>No | Hyperprolactinemia, thyroid disorders, testicular failure are common causes of impotence.<br>Vascular diseases may manifest with impotence, claudication, cold extremities and skin ulcers.<br>Surgeries like peripheral vascular surgery, colostomy often result in impotence. |
| *Do you have any allergies to plants, animals or medications?*<br>No<br>*Are you taking any other medications beside the blood pressure pills?*<br>No<br>It may not be appropriate to ask you over the phone. But, doctor, I hope you understand my situation. Could you please prescribe viagra for me?<br>*Mr.Hudson, I understand that are very anxious about your sexual performance. But I should be very systematic in dealing with your problem. First of all we must identify the exact cause of your problem. Only then will I be able to think of any prescriptions that might help you. Am I clear to you?*<br>Yes, thank you, doctor.<br><br>*Have you noticed any relationship between taking your blood pressure pills and problems with erection?*<br>I am not sure doctor | Allergies<br><br>Medications<br>Ask about medications in all patients presenting with impotence. Medications such as anticholinergics, antiandrogens, antidepressants, antipsychotics may cause impotence.<br><br><br>Do not prescribe drugs over the phone before you identify the exact cause of patient's illness.<br><br><br>Antihypertensives may cause impotence as a side effect. |
| *How are your spirits? Are you feeling happy or depressed?*<br>I am slightly depressed, doctor, because of my concerns about my erection problem. I do not want to look like a sissy to my wife. | Psychiatric history<br>Think of a psychogenic cause in all patients complaining of impotence. Depression, anxiety, psychosis are common psychiatric causes of impotence. However, most cases of male erectile |

| | |
|---|---|
| *Are you taking any drugs for depression?* No, I don't think my problem is that serious. | disorders have an organic rather than a psychogenic cause. |
| *Have you ever had a psychiatric problem?* I am perfect, doctor, never. | Antidepressants may cause impotence as a side effect. |
| *Have you ever worried about successful sexual performance before?* No | Worry about a successful performance may disturb the patient's focus on the sexual stimuli resulting in erectile dysfunction. |
| *Have you ever been hospitalized?* No, doctor | Hospitalizations To some extent history of hospitalizations help the physician to estimate the overall general health of a patient. |
| *Do you have any urinary complaints like experiencing pain while urinating?* No | Urinary complaints |
| *Do you lose urine in your clothes without your control?* No | Autonomic neuropathies may present with impotence and urinary incontinence |
| *Have you noticed any increase in frequency of urination?* No | Diabetes mellitus may present with increased urination and impotence |
| *Have you ever had a kidney disease?* No | Chronic medical illnesses like renal failure, malignancy may cause impotence. Use simple words in your questions: Kidney—not renal Liver—not hepatic Heart—not cardiac Brain—not cerebral Skin—not dermatological Hormonal—not endocrinal Cancer—not malignancy High blood pressure—not hypertension |

| | |
|---|---|
| *Have you been nauseated?*<br>No<br>*Did you feel sick to your stomach?*<br>No<br>*How are your bowel movements?*<br>Normal, I go daily | Gastrointestinal complaints<br>Diseases like diabetic neuropathy may present with both gastric symptoms and impotence. Therefore ask for any gastrointestinal problems in all patients presenting with impotence. |
| *Let me ask you some questions about your sleep. Do you have problems falling asleep, staying asleep, or waking up?*<br>No<br><br>*Have you ever had any normal erections during sleep or early morning?*<br>I am not aware, doctor | Sleep history<br>Normal men frequently awaken in the morning with an erection, which is a local response to a full bladder.<br><br>If patient reports nocturnal erections—think of a psychogenic cause of impotence<br>If patient reports no nocturnal erections—think of an organic cause of impotence. Note: It is important to remember that patient may not be aware of nocturnal erections. Therefore do not diagnose an organic cause definitively even if the patient reports no nocturnal erections |
| *Are there any illnesses that run in your family?*<br>Cancer<br>*What type of cancer?*<br>I don't know | FOSSED: Family history |
| *During one sexual encounter how many times do you try to get an erection?*<br>May be 3-4 times and I am failing every time I try to maintain my erection.<br><br>*How is the health of your partner?*<br>She is perfect<br>*Let me ask you some more confidential questions. Have you tried sex with an alternative partner?*<br>Never | Sexual history<br>Situational impotence (i.e.with one partner but not another) is good evidence of a psychological impotence. Therefore ask about patient's sexual performance at different partners.<br><br>Evidence of sexual potential with an alternative partner may an indication of psychogenic impotence where as |

| | |
|---|---|
| | persistence of problem with every partner may be due to an organic cause. |
| *Do you have any marital difficulties?*<br>No<br><br>*Ever had an STD?*<br>No | Family problems like marital difficulties and bereavement are potential causes of psychogenic impotence. |
| *Do you smoke?*<br>No<br>*Did you smoke in the past?*<br>Never | Ask SODA in social history.<br>S for Smoking<br>Tobacco consumption is associated with an increased risk of sexual dysfunction. |
| *What type of work do you do?*<br>I am a school teacher<br><br>*Do you feel any excessive stress at your job?*<br>No<br><br>*Do you have any concerns about retirement etc.?*<br>No<br><br>*Do you use any recreational drugs?*<br>Very rarely doctor, just once or twice a month.<br><br>*Which ones do you use?*<br>Heroin<br><br>*Do you drink alcohol?*<br>No, never | O for Occupation<br><br>Stress in the patient's life occasionally result in erectile dysfunction.<br><br>Job related concerns like retirement may also lead to erectile dysfunction.<br><br>D for Drugs<br>Seek for a history of substance abuse in all patients presenting with impotence. For example, heroin is one of the causes of impotence<br><br>A for Alcohol<br>Alcoholism is one of the causes of impotence. |
| *Are you involved in any type of physical activity like exercise?*<br>No | Exercise<br>Problems like claudication may be uncovered when the patient with peripheral vascular disease involves in exercises like jogging. |

| | |
|---|---|
| *Now, tell me about your diet?*<br>I eat just regular stuff, with low salt | Diet<br>Exploring dietary habits of the patient helps in recommending dietary changes. (e.g. salt restriction in hypertension, sugar restriction in diabetes, saturated fats restriction in obesity, increasing fiber intake in constipation etc) |
| *So, Mr.Hudson, you have told me that you have been troubling with maintaining erections for the last 3 months, right?*<br>Yes<br>*It started gradually and worsening constantly, right?*<br>Yes<br>*You also have high blood pressure for the last 5 years and you have been taking pills to control it. Right?*<br>Yes<br>*Mr. Hudson, I need to do a physical on you. Believe me, when you come to my office, I am not going to ask again every question I asked you over the phone. But, I need to examine your genital organs, evaluate your neurological status, strength of your muscles and condition of your blood vessels. This will help me estimate your overall health accurately and establish the cause of your sexual problem definitively.* | Summary<br>Summarize the essential features of the patient's illness at least once or twice in each patient encounter. |
| *Now, coming to your chief concern this morning, I am suspecting a number of causes. Your inability to maintain your erection for the desired time may be due to a side-effect of blood pressure medication you have been taking or due to the accident you are involved in last month or due to a problem related to your blood vessels or nerve supply. You also* | Counseling<br><br><br><br>Counsel the patient on general health, smoking cessation, substance abuse, and exercise. |

*told me that you have been taking heroin occasionally. Unfortunately, heroin is a cause of impotence in many patients.*

*We need to do some tests in order to tell you the exact cause of your problem.*

*We should measure your blood sugar level and hormones like testosterone and prolactin because diabetes and hormonal imbalances are also frequent causes of impotence. So please make an appointment to visit me as soon as possible. I want to do a physical examination on you and give you some more counseling. Finally, I encourage you to keep recording your attempts for erection, duration of erection and failures*

The cause of impotence may be multifactorial. Therefore do not give a definitive diagnosis to the patient. At this movement, explain only the differential diagnosis to the patient.

Explain the importance of medical tests you are going to order.

*Mr. Hudson, it has been showed substantially that lifestyle modification may prevent many complications of high blood pressure. Take diets rich in fruits, vegetables, low-fat diary products with reduced salt. I also advise you to stop smoking and heroin use. I will be glad to supply you with some information about support groups, who can help you stopping alcohol consumption and smoking.*

*Also consider starting an exercise program. These modifications in your life style not only decrease your chances of getting a heart disease as a complication of your high blood pressure, but also improve the quality of your sexual life.*

Encourage record keeping of patient's attempts for erection, duration of erections, and failures.

*Do you have any questions for me?*

No, doctor, thank you for your time. I will make an appointment to see you soon in your office.

Give the patient the opportunity to ask any questions

---

*That will be great, Thank you, Mr.Hudson, I look forward to see you in my office.*

Bye, bye, doctor

*Bye, bye*

Farewell

Close the patient encounter with a pleasant smile, thank you and good bye

# 6

# WRITING PATIENT NOTE

*Record what you have seen; makefff a note at the time; do not wait—*
Sir William Osler

## INTRODUCTION

After you come out of examination room after each patient encounter, you will be directed by the proctor towards a writing table, where you are required to write the patient note for that particular encounter you have just finished. However, for a few cases like pre-employment check up, you do not need to write the patient note. Simply fill the form and wait for the next patient encounter. You must finish your patient encounter—history taking and physical examination—with in fifteen minutes. Keep in mind that once you leave the patient to complete your patient note, you cannot re-enter the examination room. So make sure that you have completed your history taking and physical examination before you leave the patient.

After your 15 minute patient encounter you are required to document your findings from the history and physical examination on a separate sheet of paper. You can also type your notes on the computer instead of writing on the sheet. Whether you would like to write on the paper or type on the computer, you should decide before starting to document the patient note. After you decide whether to write or type, you are not allowed to change your decision for the documentation of that particular case:
You will be provided with a blank paper for note taking in the examination room. Note all the pertinent positives and negatives on the blank paper. Your blank paper is not scored and you can use it as you wish.

## GOLDEN RULES TO WRITE A PATIENT NOTE SUCCESSFULLY:

**Before patient encounter:**

1. **Decide before hand**, what format you are going to use to document the patient note:

Writing on the sheet or typing on the computer. Very rarely computers do not work in the examination center. In such circumstances the test center staff will ask you to write down your patient note. Therefore always be prepared to write down your patient note.

2.  Remember through your patient note—unlike history taking and physical examination—**you are communicating with another health professional**. You are the author of this note. It should reflect your thinking of patient's problem rather than writing down every word verbatim from the patient. Approach the patient note writing with this point in mind.
3.  Before you enter the examination room for patient interview you will be given a blank paper to take notes inside. **Write down the following mnemonic** on this blank paper.
    KISS RED CPR LIQOR FAAA TRIFT PAMP HUGS FOSSED

4.  Extend the social history as SODA
5.  **Note down** the last name, chief complaint, and vital signs **on your blank paper directly from the doorway information sheet** posted on the door of the patient examination room. **This saves some time** avoiding the need to visit the doorway information sheet frequently for collecting the information.

**During the patient encounter:**

1.  During the patient encounter feel free to take notes on the blank paper, which will be provided by the test center proctors. Write down the pertinent positives and negatives against the alphabet of the mnemonic. However, remember that you should take notes in a fashion that does not diminish your rapport with the patient. Tell the patient that you will be taking a few notes during the interview: *"Mr. Daniel, as our conversation moves forward, I would like to make a few notes on this sheet of paper. Is that all right with you? Thank you"*
2.  Do not try to enter everything the patient tells you. Write down only the pertinent positive and negative findings that are essential in the context of patient's present illness. Needless to say, the same information, which is useful to analyze the patient's present illness, is also necessary to write the relevant patient note.

**After the patient encounter:**

1.  Sit at your desk and start writing the patient note either by writing on the sheet provided or typing on the computer mounted on the desk. Go for typing on the computer only if your typing skills are good. Otherwise, it is better to write down on the paper.

2.  Use the notes you have taken on the blank paper as your guide to write the patient note, unless you have extraordinary memory. Document the pertinent findings on the patient note, directly from the blank paper.

3.  If you are unable to use your blank paper during the patient encounter, recap the above mnemonic, then following the alphabet of the mnemonic unleash the information and findings of the patient encounter from the memory.

4.  In an actual practice setting, the patient note would be used to communicate with other health professionals. Therefore, the note should be legible to someone other than the writer. Write legibly: write as clearly as possible; it should be easily read with little effort required.

5.  Group similar data together in a logical sequence. Write out information in a logical sequence

6.  Document significant positive and negative elements of the history and physical examination with appropriate detail. Identifying critical elements is also important.

7.  Be specific, use precise descriptions of physical findings and avoid vague terms such as "Clear" or "OK"

8.  Sometimes it is necessary to record the findings just as they are described than through your interpretation. For example, a patient described that he felt his chest pain as if someone stabbed him with a long knife and twisted it in his chest. It is better to record it as, "Patient described his chest pain as, "someone stabbing me with a long knife and twisting it in my chest", not as, 'Patient described his chest pain in violent terms' or 'patient described his chest pain in a bizarre fashion'

9.  Your differential diagnosis should reflect the interpretation of data gathered from the patient's history and physical examination. This requirement discourages concocting a 'textbook differential diagnosis' of a particular condition. Identify critical elements which help you to form the differential diagnosis.

10.  Diagnostic work up should be consistent with differential diagnosis. The tests you order should be reasonable and appropriate to the patient's condition.

11.  Avoid diagnostic work up plans that could result in harm.

12.  Avoid expensive, non-indicated diagnostic tests.

13.  Do not include treatment plans or referrals or hospitalizations in your patient note.

14.  Use well known abbreviations to save both time and space. If you are doubtful about any abbreviation write down the word in full.

---

**Do not write prescriptions or treatment plans in your patient note**
Patient: Doctor, what I need is something to stir me up; something to put me in a fighting mood. Did you put something like that in this prescription?
Doctor: No need for that. You will find that in your bill.☺

---

# ABBREVIATIONS

Try to learn the following abbreviations to save both time and space on patient note. Use only the abbreviations, which are common enough to be recognized by all doctors. If you have any doubt about an abbreviation, it is better to write it in words.

**Units of measures:**

Kg—Kilogram
g—Gram
mg—Milligram
lbs—Pounds
oz—Ounces
m—Meter
cm—Centimeter
min—Minute
hr—Hour
C—Centigrade
F—Fahrenheit

**Vital Signs**

BP—Blood pressure
HR—Heart Rate
R—Respirations
T—Temperature
yo Year-old
m or ♂ Male
f or ♀ Female
b black
w white
L Left
R Right
hx History
h/o History of
c/o Complaining of
NL Normal limits
WNL within normal limits
+ positive
—negative

## Other Abbreviations

AA—Alcoholics Anonymous; African American

AAA—Abdominal Aortic Aneurysm

ABD—Abdomen

ABG—Arterial Blood Gas

ABPA—Allergic Broncho Pulmonary Aspergillosis

ABX—Antibiotics

ACE-I—Angiotensin Converting Enzyme Inhibitor

ACL—Anterior Cruciate Ligament

ADD—Attention Deficit Disorder

ADE—Adverse Drug Effect

ADHD—Attention Deficit Hyperactivity Disorder

ADL—Activities of Daily Living

ADR—Adverse Drug Reaction

AF—Atrial Fibrillation

AFB—Acid Fast Bacterium

AFP—Alpha Fetoprotein

AGN—Antigen

AIDS—Acquired Immuno-Deficiency Syndrome

AKA—Above Knee Amputation

ALS—Amyotrophic Lateral Sclerosis

AMI—Acute Myocardial Infarction; Anterior Myocardial Infarction

A&O—Alert And Oriented

AP—Anterior-Posterior

APPY—Appendectomy

ARDS—Adult Respiratory Distress Syndrome

ARF—Acute Renal Failure

AS—Aortic Stenosis

ASA—Aspirin

ATN—Acute Tubular Necrosis

B—Bilateral

BAE—Barium Enema

BCC—Basal Cell Carcinoma

BCG—Bacille Calmette-Guerin

BID—Twice a Day

BKA—Below Knee Amputation

BL CX—Blood Culture

BM—Bone Marrow; also Bowel Movement

BMI—Body Mass Index

BMT—Bone Marrow Transplant

BP—Blood Pressure

BPV—Benign Positional Vertigo
BS—Bowel Sounds; Breath Sounds; Blood Sugar
BSA—Body Surface Area
BUN—Blood Urea Nitrogen
BX—Biopsy
C—With
CABG—Coronary Artery By-Pass Graft
CAD—Coronary Artery Disease
CATH—Catheterization
C/B—Complicated By
CBC—Complete Blood Count
CBD—Common Bile Duct
CC—Chief Complaint
CCU—Cardiac care unit
Cig—Cigarettes
CCB—Calcium Channel Blocker
CCK—Cholycystectomy
CCE—Clubbing, Cyanosis, Edema
C/D—Cup to Disk ratio
C DIF—Clostridium Difficile
CEA—Carcinoembryonic Antigen
Chemo—Chemotherapy
CHI—Closed Head Injury
CHF—Congestive Heart Failure
Choly—Cholycystectomy
CI—Cardiac Index
CK—Creatine Kinase
CL—Chloride
CLL—Chronic Lymphocytic Leukemia
CM—Cardiomegaly
CML—Chronic Myelogenous Leukemia
CMP—Cardiomyopathy
CMT—Cervical Motion Tenderness
CMV—Cyto-Megalo Virus
CN—Cranial Nerves
CNS—Central Nervous System
CO—Cardiac Output
C/O—Complains Of
COPD—Chronic Obtructive Pulmonary Disease
COX 2—Cyclooxygenase 2
CPR—Cardiopulmonary Resuscitation
CRVO—Central Retinal Vein Occlusion

CSF—Cerebral Spinal Fluid
CT—Computerized tomography
CTA—Clear To Auscultation
CVA or—Cerebral Vascular Accident
TIA—Transient ischemic attack
CVP—Central Venous Pressure
C/W—Consistent with
CX—Culture
CXR—Chest X-Ray
DB—Direct Bilirubin
D&C—Dilatation and Curettage
DF—Dorsiflexion
DI—Diabetes Insipidus;
Detrusor Instability
DIC—Disseminated Intravascular Coagulopathy
DIF—Differential
DIP—Distal Inter-Phalangeal
DJD—Degenerative Joint Disease
DKA—Diabetic Ketoacidosis
DM—Diabetes Mellitus
D/O—Disorder
DP—Dorsalis Pedis
DR—Diabetic Retinopathy
DRE—Digital Rectal Exam
D/T—Due To
DTs—Delirium Tremens
DTR—Deep Tendon Reflex
DVT—Deep Venous Thrombosis
DX—Diagnosis
DU—Duodenal Ulcer
EBV—Epstein Barr Virus
ECG—Electrocardiogram (also known as EKG)
ECHO—Echocardiography
ECMO—Extra-Corporeal Membrane Oxygenation
ECT—Electro-Convulsive Therapy
ED—Erectile Dysfunction; Emergency Department
EEG—Electroencephalogram
EGD—Esophago-Gastro Duodenoscopy
EJ—External Jugular
EM—Electron Microscopy
EMG—Electromyelogram
EMT—emergency medical technician

ENT—ear, nose, and throat
EOMI—Extra Ocular Muscles Intact
ER—External Rotation; Emergency Room
ERCP—Endoscopic Retrograde Cholangio-Pancreotography
ESLD—End Stage Liver Disease
ESR—Erythrocyte Sedimentation Rate
ESRD—End Stage Renal Disease
ESWL—Extracorporeal Shock Wave Lithotripsy
ETOH—Alcohol
EX LAP—Exploratory Laparotomy
EX FIX—External Fixation
Ext.—Extremities
FB—Foreign Body
F/B—Followed By
FBS—Fasting Blood Sugar
Fe—Iron
Fem—Femoral
FENa—Fractional Excretion of Sodium
FEV1—Forced Expiratory Volume 1 Second
FH—Family history
FNA—Fine Needle Aspiration
FOOSH—Fall On Outstretched Hand
FP—Family Practitioner
FRC—Functional Residual Capacity
FSG—Finger Stick Glucose
FSH—Follicle Stimulating Hormone
FTT—Failure To Thrive
F/U—Follow-Up
FUO—Fever of Unknown Origin
Fx—Fracture
G—Guiac (followed by + or- )
GAD—Generalized Anxiety Disorder
GB—Gall Bladder
GBM—Glioblastoma Multiforme
GBS—Group B Strep
GC—Gonorrhea
GERD—Gastroesophageal Reflux
GI—Gastrointestinal
GIB—Gastrointestinal Bleeding
GLC—Glaucoma
GMR—Gallups, Murmurs, Rubs
GOO—Gastric Outlet Obstruction

G#P#—Gravida # Para #

GSW—Gun Shot Wound

GTT—Glucose Tolerance Test

GU—Genito-Urinary; also Gastric Ulcer

GVHD—Graft Versus Host Disease

H FLU—Haemophilus Influenza

HA—Headache

HACE—High Altitude Cerebral Edema

HAPE—High Altitude Pulmonary Edema

HCC—Hepatocellular Carcinoma

HCG—Human Chorionic Gonadotropin

HCT—Hematocrit

HCV—Hepatitis C Virus

HD—Hemodialysis

HDL—High Density Lipoprotein

HEENT—Head, Ears, Eyes, Nose, Throat

HGB—Hemoglobin

HH—Hiatal Hernia

H&H—Hemoglobin and Hematocrit

HI—Homicidal Ideation

HIB—Haemophilus Influenza B vaccine

HIT—Heparin Induced Thrombocytopenia

HIV—Human Immunodeficiency Virus

HOCM—Hypertrophic Obstructive Cardiomyopathy

HPI—History of Present Illness

HPV—Human Papilloma Virus

HR—Heart Rate

HRT—Hormone Replacement Therapy

HS—At Bedtime

HSM—Holo-Systolic Murmur; also Hepato-Splenomegaly

HSP—Henoch Schonlein Purpura

HSV—Herpes Simplex Virus

HTN—Hypertension

HUS—Hemolytic Uremic Syndrome

HX—History

IBD—Inflammatory Bowel Disease

IBS—Irritable Bowel Syndrome

ICH—Intra-Cranial Hemorrhage

ICP—Intra-Cranial Pressure

ID—Infectious Diseases

I&D—Incise and Drain

IDDM—Insulin Dependent Diabetes Mellitus

IFN—Interferon

IH—Inguinal Hernia (usually preceded by L or R)

IJ—Internal Jugular

ILD—Interstitial Lung Disease

IMI—Inferior Myocardial Infarction

IP—Inter-Phalangeal

IR—Internal Rotation

ITP—Idiopathic Thrombocytopenia

IUD—Intrauterine Device

IUP—Intrauterine Pregnancy

IV—Intravenous

IVC—Inferior Vena Cava

IVDU—Intravenous Drug Use

IVF—Intravenous Fluids; also In Vitro Fertilization

IVP—Intravenous Pyelogram

JVD—Jugular Venous Distention

JVP—Jugular Venous Pressure

K—Potassium

Kcal—Kilocalories

KUB—Kidneys, Ureters and Bladder

L—Left

LA—Left Atrium

LAC—Laceration

LAP—Laparoscopic; also Laparotomy

LBBB—Left Bundle Branch Block

LBO—Large Bowel Obstruction

LBP—Low Back Pain

LCL—Lateral Collateral Ligament

L&D—Labor and Delivery

LDH—Lactate Dehydrogenase

LDL—Low Density Lipoprotein

LFT—Liver Function Test

LH—Leutinizing hormone

LMN—Lower Motor Neuron

LMP—Last Menstrual Period

LOC—Loss Of Consciousness

LP—Lumbar Puncture

LS—Lumbo-Sacral

LT—Light Touch

MCP—Metacarpal-Phalangeal

MCV—Mean Corpuscular Volume

MDRTB—Multi-Drug Resistant Tuberculosis

MI—Myocardial Infarction
MM—Multiple Myeloma
MMR—Measles, Mumps and Rubella vaccine
MRI—Magnetic Resonance Imaging
MRSA—Methicillin Resistant Staph Aureus
MTP—Metatarsal-Phalangeal
MVA—motor vehicle accident
MVP—Mitral Valve Prolapse
MVR—Mitral Valve Replacement
N—Nausea
NAD—No Apparent Distress; No Acute Disease
NABS—Normal Active Bowel Sounds
NCAT—Normocephalic Atraumatic
NCS—Nerve Conduction Study
Neuro—Neurologic
NIDDM—Non-Insulin Dependent Diabetes Mellitus
NKA—No Known Allergies
NKDA—No Known Drug Allergies
NMS—Neuroleptic Malignant Syndrome
NOS—Not Otherwise Specified
NSR—Normal Sinus Rhythm
NT—Non-Tender
OA—Osteoarthritis
OB—Occult Blood (followed by '+' or '-')
OCD—Obsessive Compulsive Disorder
OCP—Oral Contraceptive Pill
OE—Otitis Externa
OM—Otitis Media
OSA—Obstructive Sleep Apnea
OTC—Over The Counter
OU—Both Eyes
O/W—Otherwise
P—Pulse
PA—Posterior-Anterior
PAD—Peripheral Arterial Disease
PBC—Primary Biliary Cirrhosis
PC—After Meals
PCKD—Polycystic Kidney Disease
PCL—Posterior Cruciate Ligament
PCOD—Poly-Cystic Ovarian Disease
PCR—Polymerase Chain Reaction
PDA—Patent Ductus Arteriosus

PE—Physical Exam
PEG—Percutaneous Endoscopic Gastrostomy
PERRLA—Pupils Equal, Round, Reactive to Light and Accommodation
PET—Positron Emission Tomography
PFTs—Pulmonary Function Tests
PID—Pelvic Inflammatory Disease
PIH—Pregnancy Induced Hypertension
PIP—Proximal Inter-Phalangeal
PMH—Past Medical History
PMI—Point of Maximum Impulse
PNA—Pneumonia
PNBX—Prostate Needle Biopsy
PND—Paroxysmal Nocturnal dyspnea
po—orally
PPD—Purified Protein Derivative
PPH—Primary Pulmonary Hypertension
PR—Per Rectum
PSA—Prostate Specific Antigen
PSC—Primary Sclerosing Cholangitis
PSH—Past Surgical History
PT—Prothrombin Time
PTCA—Percutaneous Transluminal Coronary Angioplasty
PTSD—Post-Traumatic Stress Disorder
PTT—Partial Thromboplastin Time
PTX—Pneumothorax
PUD—Peptic Ulcer Disease
PV—Polycythemia Vera; Portal Vein
RBBB—Right Bundle Branch Block
RBC—Red Blood Cell
RCC—Renal Cell Cancer
RD—Retinal Detachment
RHD—Rheumatic Heart Disease
Rheum—Rheumatology
ROM—Range Of Motion
ROS—Review Of Systems
RPGN—Rapidly Progressive Glomerulonephritis
RPLND—Retroperitoneal Lymph Node Dissection
RR—Respiratory Rate
RRR—Regular Rate and Rhythm
RSD—Reflex Sympathetic Dystrophy
RSV—Respiratory Syncytial Virus
RUQ—Right Upper Quadrant

S—Without

2/2—Secondary To

SAB—Spontaneous Abortion

SAH—Sub-Arachnoid Hemorrhage

SBE—Subacute Bacterial Endocarditis

SBO—Small Bowel Obstruction

SBP—Spontaneous Bacterial Peritonitis; Systolic Blood Pressure

SC—Subcutaneous

SI—Suicidal Ideation

SIADH—Syndrome of Inappropriate Anti-Diuretic Hormone secretion

SIDS—Sudden Infant Death Syndrome

SLE—Systemic Lupus Erythematosus

SLR—Straight Leg Raise

STD—Sexually Transmitted Disease

STS—Soft Tissue Swelling

STX—Stricture

SW—Stab Wound

SX—Symptoms

SZR—Seizure

T—Temperature

T&A—Tonsillectomy and Adenoidectomy

TAA—Thoracic Aortic Aneurysm

TAB—Threatened Abortion; also Therapeutic Abortion

TAH—Total Abdominal Hysterectomy

TB—Tuberculosis; Total Bilirubin

TEE—Trans-Esophageal Echocardiogram

TIA—Transient Ischemic Attack

TIBC—Total Iron Binding Capacity

TID—Three times per day

TIPS—Transvenous Intrahepatic Porto-Systemic Shunt

TKA—Total Knee Arthroplasty

TKR—Total Knee Replacement

TMJ—Temporo-Mandibular Joint

TOA—Tubo-Ovarian Abscess

TOX—Toxicology

TOXO—Toxoplasmosis

TP—Total Protein

TPN—Total Parenteral Nutrition

TR—Tricuspid Regurgitation

TRUS—Transrectal Ultrasound

T&S—Type and Screen

TSH—Thyroid Stimulating Hormone

U/A—Urinalysis
UC—Ulcerative Colitis
UCX—Urine Culture
UMN—Upper Motor Neuron
UNSA—Unstable Angina
UO—Urine Output
URI—Upper Respiratory tract Infection
US—Ultrasound
UTD—Up To Date
UTI—Urinary Tract Infection
UV—Ultraviolet
V—Vomiting
VA—Visual Acuity
VAX—Vaccine
VBAC—Vaginal Birth After Cesarean Section
VF—Ventricular Fibrillation
VS—Vital Signs
VSD—Ventricular Septal Defect
VT—Ventricular Tachycardia
VWF—Von Willebrand Factor
WBC—White Blood Cells
WDWN—Well Developed, Well Nourished
WNL—Within Normal Limits
W/O—Without
W/U—Work-Up
X—Except
XLR—Crossed Leg Raise
ZE—Zollinger-Ellision syndrome

# COMMON TO ALL CASES

Many students find it difficult to put their thoughts into words even after a vigorous patient encounter. Following examples are given so that the student can become more familiar with common medical write-up and become more comfortable in recording the medical data.

## CHIEF COMPLAINT

**Chief complaint should be recorded in the patient's own words**

Mr. John Friedman is a 46-year old white male came with a complaint of "I could not tolerate this belly pain"

Mrs. Josephine Christopher is a 29-year old black female, who has a history of diabetes since 1994, came here for medication refill

Mrs. Rosemary Church, mother of 1 year-old baby John Church, came in because, "her son is pooping without stopping"

Mr. Daniel Johnson is 56-year old male complaing of "pretty yucky headaches"

Mr. Frances Fleming is a 75 year-old white female who came because of 'bumps on her right leg'

## HISTORY OF PRESENT ILLNESS

This is a 36-year-old white woman was normal until this morning, when she developed a vague abdominal pain. The pain was initially localized on periumbilical region and then, within 12 hours, moved to being well localized on the right lower quadrant. The pain is increasing with walking or coughing. The patient had nausea and two episodes of vomiting in the last two hours. She has a sense of constipation associated with a low grade fever.

This is a 62 year-old white male, who was well until two hours ago, suddenly developed severe chest pain while reading newspaper after getting up from the bed. Though the patient has a history of anginal attacks, he complains that this pain is more severe and radiating into his left arm. The pain is not relieved by Nitroglycerin. He also refers to having dyspnea, a cold sweat, weakness, wheezing, and nausea and vomiting.

This is a 25-year-old male, who presents to the emergency room with symptoms of retrosternal discomfort, not associate with nausea or vomiting. Patient states that he was using cannabis over the weekend and developed some abdominal discomfort and nausea, this persisted over the weekend, but he felt better on Monday. However yesterday he noticed some retrosternal discomfort and hence he came up to the emergency room. Patient denies any exertion dyspnea, orthopnea, or PND. No exertional chest pain.

This is a 40-year-old-male who had onset of migraines 6-7 years ago and she had a prior migraine for the first time at age 18. She states that she was getting worse. She has a retro-orbital pain, which is associated with a steady, aching pain up to 10/10 when severe, but the average is mild to moderate ranging from 2/10 to 4/10. She wakes up in the morning with headaches. The headaches can last from 1-3 days. She often has nausea associated with her headaches, emesis, photophobia, and phonophobia and has to sleep in a dark room to feel better. She states that her migraines are not associated with an aura. She is having approximately 3 headaches per day.

HPI: An 87-year-old white male with a history of right groin and bilateral knee pain that started yesterday; got worse and could not stand or walk like he usually does. Denies any trauma or fall. Pain does not radiate;no numbness or tingling. Also has chronic bilateral leg ulcers. Sees the Wound Clinic; was supposed to be on antibiotics, but has not been taking.The patient received Levaquin 500 mg IV in the emergency room.

## REVIEW OF SYSTEMS

ROS: The patient denies any fever or chills. Denies cold, sore throat, exertional dyspnea, orthopnea or PND. The patient denies any dysuria or hematuria. Gastrointestinal symptoms as in the HPI. Patient denies any focal limb weakness or easy bruising. No history of polyuria or polydipsia. No allergies. Denies any depression or anxiety.

| | |
|---|---|
| General: | some weight gain over a period of 5 years. She gained 30 lbs. |
| HEENT: | Headaches as stated above |
| CVS: | negative, no chest pain |
| Respiratory system: | negative, no shortness of breath |
| GI: | History of bloody urine for which she has had extensive work-up with no known etiology for this problem per patient |
| Psychiatric: | Negative |

| | |
|---|---|
| HEENT: | Normal |
| Respiratory: | cough with occasional sputum production |
| Cardiac: | palpitations |
| GI: | Normal |
| Renal/GU: | pain associated with micturition, referring to the distal urethra |

| | |
|---|---|
| ROS: | Unremarkable. |

| | |
|---|---|
| Constitutional: | Negative for chills, fatigue, fever, and weight change |
| Eyes: | Negative for blurred vision, eye pain, and photophobia |
| ENT: | Negative for hearing problems, ENT pain, congestion, rhinorrhea, epistaxis, hoarseness, and dental problems |
| CVS: | Positive for palpitations. Negative for chest pain, claudication, paroxysmal nocturnal dyspnea, pedal edema, tachycardia, or varicosities. |

| | |
|---|---|
| Respiratory: | Negative for cough, dyspnea, and hemoptysis |
| Gastrointestinal: | Negative for abdominal pain, heartburn, constipation, diarrhea, and stool changes |
| Genitourinary: | Negative for genital lesions, hematuria, menstrual problems, polyuria, abnormal vaginal bleeding, and vaginal discharge. |

Neurological:     Negative for dizziness, headaches, paresthesias, and weakness
Endocrine:        Negative for hair loss, heat/cold intolerance, polydipsia. And
                  polyphagia.

**Location:** For all pain complaints, use LIQOR FAAA TRIFT as the guide to document the history in the patient note.

Pain located in the right costovertebral angle.
The chest pain is felt behind or slightly to the left of the mid sternum.
The pain was felt initially in the lower jaw, the back of the neck and then the interscapular area.
Foreign body sensation in the right eye.

## Intensity
Pain score 0/10
Pain is average to mild ranging from 2/10 to 4/10

## Quality
Squeezing, burning, and pressing pain
Patient complains of a low, midline, wave-like, cramping pelvic pain radiating to inner thighs.
Burning and stinging pain in the perianal skin and the buttocks.
Steady, boring and severe pain in the epigastrium.

## Onset and duration
Patient reports a sudden, severe, lancinating, intermittent pain in the lower quadrant.

## Radiation
Pain is radiating from costovertebral angle to the umbilicus.
Pain is referring to the right testicle from the right costovertebral angle.
Pain is referring to the left labium from the left costovertebral angle.
Pain is referring to the scrotum from the right lower quadrant.
Pain is radiating from the scrotum to the right groin.

## Frequency
Pain comes appro.4 times per day

## Aggravating factors
Patient complains of an epigastric abdominal pain, abrupt in onset, and aggravated by walking and lying supine and relieved by sitting and leaning forward.
Patient reports the breast pain increases during premenstrual phase of cycle.
Aggravating factors include weight-bearing.

**Alleviating factors**
Patient complains of knee pain made worse by activity or weight bearing and relieved by rest.

**Associated factors**
Associated symptoms include swelling and bruising, but not crepitus or ankle instability.

**Trauma**
The precipitating event appears to have been hit leg against her fridge.

**Rash**
Rash appeared on the fifth day of fever on the wrists and ankles and then spread centrally.

**Infections/Insect bites**
Patient remembers begin bitten by a tick during his last vacation in the woods of California.

**Fever**
Patient complains of an evening rise of temperature for the last 11 days.
Patient feels hotter than usual but not sure that she has been running a fever.

**Travel**
Patient states that he traveled to Kenya two months ago without taking malaria prophylaxis.
Patient states that he went to Mexico for the summer vacation and remembers that he drank water from unprotected sources two times.
Patient told that he went to Bangladesh to visit his relatives and spending two days in the home of a relative, who has tuberculosis.
Writing all pain characteristics in one sentence:

ROS:

Positive for weight change, No fever. No night sweats, No change in vision, No change in hearing, No cough, No shortness of breath, No chest pain, No palpitations, Positive edema, No abdominal pain, No vomiting, No change in bowel habits, No dysuria, No hematuria. Positive joint pain of the right shoulder. Positive history of trauma. No frequent headaches

**Past Medical History**
Past medical history: None significant
There is no past medical history of hypertension, diabetes, tuberculosis, sexually transmitted disease, stroke or heart disease.
He was diagnosed with hypertension in 1992 and MI in 1999.

She was diagnosed with Type-2 Diabetes Mellitus in 1985; treated with weight reduction through diet and exercise until 1994; Then she was on oral medications— Sulfonylureas and repaglinide for 4 years, after which she was switched to insulin injections.

She had a total hysterectomy about 12 years ago, and headaches as stated above. The patient has a history of questionable seizure and loss of consciousness 5-6 years ago. She had an MRI done at the time of brain which was normal. She does not recall having an EEG, but this episode did not recur.

Past Medical history: Atrial fibrillation in 2001, peptic ulcer disease in 2008

Past Medical History: Non-small cell lung cancer diagnosed 08/07 involving the right lung. He has extensive adenopathy and was staged T1 N3.

## Past surgical History

Appendectomy 1996

Coronary artery bypass surgery, 1991

Angioplasty, 1995; Total hysterectomy, April 1997

Patient has a history of left medial meniscal injury, 1996, with subsequent surgical repair.

Benign colonic adenomatous polyps removed on screening colonoscopy, 6/98, 10/99.

Surgical history: None

Surgical history:

Hysterectomy

Tonsillectomy

Past surgical history: no previous surgeries

## Allergies

Allergies:   None known

Allergies:   allergic to neomycin and diphenylhydramine.

Allergies:   no known drug allergies. Although she has a side effect to codeine with increased nausea.

Allergies:   Patient admits allergies to codeine

## Medications

Medications: None

Medications: Loperamide 2 mg after each loose stool

Ciprofloxacin 750 mg OD

Medications: Patient uses vitamins but does not routinely use prescription medications.

Immunizations are current

Patient complains of headache, nasopharyngitis, and upper respiratory infection since starting his treatment with valacyclovir, 500mg per day, three weeks ago.

Current medications:

1.  Hydrocodone 2 tablets p.o.p.r.n. She is taking 8 times per week
2.  ESGIC 1 t.i.d to q.i.d.
3.  Flexeril 10 mg 2 p.o.q.h.s.

Current medications: Lanoxin and Coumadin
Current medications: She has been taking some Darvocet without much help.

## Psychiatric History:
She was diagnosed with Schizophrenia in 1993; attempted suicide in 1996.
Patient has a history of Obsessive Compulsive Disorder since 2001

## Hospitalizations
Patient was hospitalized a month ago for the treatment of pneumonia, which lasted for a week.
Her only hospitalization was in 1996 for appendectomy

## Urological symptoms
Patient complains of increased frequency, intense thirst, especially a craving for ice water.
Patient has recurrent episodes of right CVA pain radiating into the right flank and groin. This come in waves and was quite steady. No position was comfortable. This was not associated with any obvious hematuria or dysuria. She has had no fever or chills.

## Gastrointestinal symptoms
She was a little nauseated but this has now passed.
She has also had diarrhea which she describes as 1-2 loose to liquid stools. Denies blood or mucus in the stool.

## Sleep pattern
Patient complains of difficulty getting to sleep, staying asleep, early morning awakening associated with intermittent wakefulness during the night
Patient complains of restless sleep, snoring, excessive daytime sleepiness associated with memory impairment and headaches.

## Family history
Father: Died of myocardial infarction at age 74
Mother: Alive and well
Brother: Age 51, diagnosed with Multiple Myeloma.

Father: 49 yo, alive and well
Mother: 48 yo, breast cancer treated by total mastectomy at age 39.

Her daughter has a history of headaches. Her grandparents have a history of cardiac problems, MI. Her mother and her grandmother had a stroke, and one of her grandfathers died of cancer at a young age, probably lung cancer.

Family history: Unremarkable

FH: Patient admits a family history of arthritis associated with father, mother.
MGM (d.age 50s), unknown cause
PGF (69), prostate cancer
MGF (d.age 87), unknown cancer
(MGM: maternal grandmother, PGF: paternal grandfather, MGF: maternal grandfather)

## Obstetric History/Gynecologic history
Patient complains of feelings of intense heat over trunk and face, with sweating and flushing of the skin, remarkably during hot weather.
Patient had irregular menstrual cycles from age 14 to 17.
Patient complains of painful intercourse for the last 2 months.
Patient complains of menstrual disturbances, purulent cervical discharge, fever, chills and lower abdominal pain.

## Sexual history
Before diagnosed with HIV, Patient had been practicing unprotected anal intercourse with his roommate since 1995.
Patient had a Pap smear last month and was told that the results were within normal limits, but that she had a slight inflammation.
Patient has her husband as the only sexual partner and he regularly uses condoms.

## Smoking
Smoking: An occasional cigar
Smoking: One pack per day for the last 16 years.
Smoking history: Patient admits tobacco use. She relates a smoking history of 40 pack years.

## Occupation:
He works as a consultant in a federal company. He has not missed work due to illness since his last physical exam.
The patient is a Vietnam veteran and states that he was exposed to Agent Orange in the Vietnam War.

## Drugs

Caffeine: Diet sodas and coffee

Inhaling heroin for the last 3 years.

Injecting Phencyclidine twice a week on the left forearm. He also states that this addiction is leading him to violent behavior.

The patient has been inhaling Marijuana by smoking on a daily basis.

Patient states that he was using cannabis over the weekend and developed some abdominal discomfort and nausea, which persisted over the weekend, but he felt better on Monday.

## Domestic violence

The patient has been a victim of domestic abuse for the last 9 months and has the evidence of posttraumatic stress disorder.

This elderly patient states that she is being abused by her caregiver in the hospice for the last 2 years.

The girl states that she is being sexually molested by her step-father several times after her mother's recent marriage with the latter.

## Alcohol:

Alcohol: None

Patient has a history of alcohol intake immediately preceding the attack.

Patient has a history of episodes of acute pancreatitis, often related to alcohol intake.

Uses alcohol; she drinks scotch; 2 drinks/day for the last 16 years

Patient is a schoolteacher. Denies tobacco or alcohol use. Gives a history of marijuana use. Denies intravenous drug abuse and denies cocaine use.

She is married, she has a daughter, she is not working, she is a housewife

No tobacco, no alcohol, no drugs

Denies smoking and ETOH

## Exercise

The patient currently runs (on average) 4.0 miles, 5 times weekly. He also routinely cross-trains with swimming, free weights, and elliptical trainer.

The patient has a history of activity and sports-related injuries. These injuries resolved without sequelae, and do not impact his current exercise program or duties.

## Diet:

Patient has been on fat-restricted diet since he was diagnosed with fat malabsorption syndrome in 1987.

Patient has been taking protein-restricted diet since he was diagnosed with hepatic encephalopathy due to chronic liver disease

**Physical Examination:** Begin physical examination with a statement about the patient's general appearance and then continue with the results of the vital signs and the results of the examination of skin, head, eyes, ears, nose, throat, neck, chest, back, heart, abdomen, extremities, musculoskeletal system, nervous system, and mental status.

# GENERAL EXAMINATION

First, make a brief comment about the patient's general appearance

**General Examination:**
Well built, well nourished, no apparent distress observed.
Mildly ill appearing and moderately distressed
Mildly ill appearing, anxious, irritable, uncooperative and alcohol on breath
Well-built, oriented, calm, and cooperative
Ill built, appears pale in the face, conjunctiva, and mucous membranes, saliva drooling from
    the mouth, has a poorly modulated voice and variable rest tremor in both hands.
Mildly disoriented, hyperactive
Patient has a relatively immobile face with fixity of facial expression, widened palpebral
    fissures, and infrequent blinking.
Patient appears frightened and fatigued
Patient is awake and alert. He is afebrile. The JVD is normal. The blood pressure is
    130/80. Pulse is 78 per minute. There is no peripheral edema, clubbing, cyanosis,
    or lymphadenopathy.
She is pleasant and cooperative with the examination.
General: well developed and nourished; appropriately groomed; in no apparent distress
General: Patient is pleasant, 55 year old female in no apparent distress who looks her given
    age, is well developed and nourished with good attention to hygiene and body habitus.

**Vital Signs:** Second, report abnormal vital signs, e.g. Temperature, blood pressure, pulse and respiratory rate. To avoid going to the doorway information sheet again and again, write down the vital signs on your blank paper before you enter the patient room.

| | |
|---|---|
| Age: | 62 years |
| Height: | 74 inches (without shoes) |
| Temperature: | 98 degrees F (oral) |
| Weight: | 186.75 |
| Heart rate: | 69 bpm |
| Blood pressure: | 119/78 |
| Pulse: | weakening of pulse during inspiration |

T 98 F, BP 150/80, P 78, R 16
T: 37.5°C, BP: 125/90 mm Hg, P: 98/min, R: 16/min

T: 38°C, BP: 140/95 mm Hg, P: 85/min, R: 18/min
Stable, T: 98.2 F, BP: 100/64 mm Hg, P: 78/min, R: 20/min

# SKIN

## HISTORY

Patient complains painful red nodules on the anterior aspect of his left leg.

Patient complains about dry plaques on the scalp

She reports dryness of skin, balding, increased muscularity, deepening of voice, and enlargement of clitoris.

Three small lesions resembling actinic keratoses were noted on the dorsal surface of right elbow.

Patient complains fever, malaise, and chills associated with a red spot appeared near a fissure at the angle of the nose

Patient states that the color of the mole has changed from beige to dark brown

Patient states that the dark spot with irregular borders, present on the right palm, has changed its color recently

She complains of hyperpigmentation of face, which was noticed five months after starting the oral contraceptive therapy.

Dependent rubor is prominent on the left leg.

Patient states the interdigital webs on the left hand are itching, burning and stinging.

Patient complains burning and itching on the trunk in hot, moist climates.

Patient complains that she has developed this callosity since wearing her new high-heeled shoes.

Patient complains of a rash that appeared first in the axillas, over the trunk and the spreading to the extremities.

Patient complains of a rash that appeared between days 2 and 6 of fever, first on the wrists and ankles, and then spreading centrally to the arms, legs, and trunk for 2-3 days.

## PHYSICAL EXAMINATION OF SKIN

Loss of hair is observed, with thinning of the skin and subcutaneous tissues, and diminution in the size of the muscles.

Skin is cool, hairless and atrophic

Pitting is observed on the nails of the right hand and nail plate of the right index finger is separated from the bed.

The left index finger is clubbed.

Nails are thin and brittle.

A rash at the waistline appears to be related to the clothing waistbands.

A brick-red, irregular, blotchy maculopapular rash on the trunk and extremities, including the palms and soles.

A macular rash in the axillas and over the trunk

A dome-shaped, umbilicated papule is found on the lower abdomen

Four cigarette burns are noted on the lateral surface of the right middle finger and the medical surface of the right index finger.

Tiny 'table salt crystals' on the dull red mucous membranes of the cheeks and on inner conjunctival folds.

IV drug needle marks are noted on the ventral surface of the left forearm

The skin over the face, neck and upper trunk is dry, leathery, and hyperpigmented

A flat brown spot with smooth borders observed on the dorsum of the left hand.

Irregular ulceration is observed on the medial aspect of the left lower leg above the malleolus

A soft corn is observed on the proximal portion of the fourth toe of the right leg.

A vaccination scar is noted over the deltoid region of the right arm.

A 3 mm, pink, well-circumscribed lesion located on the right cheek

Two blue-black patches are observed on the shins

Bronze colored skin pigmentation on the upper part of the body.

Skin is dark, dry and scaly.

Skin is warm and dry and pink with moist mucous membranes.

# HEAD

**HISTORY**

Patient complains of dull, lateralized headache associated with anorexia, nausea, vomiting, photophobia, phonophobia and blurring of vision

Patient reports a headache that is worse on arising in the morning

**PHYSICAL EXAMINATION**

Head: Normocephalic, atraumatic and free of visible lesions

Head: Normocephalic, atraumatic and no evidence of head trauma

# EYES

**HISTORY**

The patient complains blurred vision with halos around lights.

The patient complains that he sees spots before the eyes associated flashing lights.

Patient complains of blurred vision progressive over three months.

Patient says that a curtain came down over her left eye, upon waking this morning

Double vision in the right eye with left eye covered

The patient complains irritation, burning and itching in the right eye

Patient complains of 'something hitting his left eye' while hammering on metal this afternoon.

The patient presented with photophobia, pain, tearing, and reduced vision

Patient complains of sensation of a foreign body in the right eye with blinking.

## PHYSICAL EXAMINATION OF EYES

Eyes: Conjunctivae clear without abnormalities, EOM intact, PERLA, no fundoscopic abnormalities, no papilledema

Vision is good and the patient wears reading glasses on an as needed basis. Ropy discharge from the left eye associated with itching is noted.

The right eye is red, with predominantly circumcorneal injection and purulent discharge.

Tenderness, redness, and swelling observed in the tear sac area.

The patient has a red eye, steamy cornea and a dilated pupil.

Sclera clear, exposed more superiorly with a widened palpebral apeture.

The conjunctiva is clear without any abnormalities.

The conjunctiva is red and elevated.

There is a hard, non-tender swelling on the right upper eye lid.

The lower lid of left eye turned outward

There is a yellow elevated nodule on the nasal side of the cornea

Gray-green ring in the cornea, most marked at the superior and inferior poles of the cornea, close to the endothelial surface.

EYES: EOMI, PERRLA; normal lids, conjunctiva, and fundoscopic exam

# EARS

## HISTORY

Patient complains of bilateral hearing loss since his air travel a week ago.

Mild hearing loss in left ear observed after completion of the instructions class in SCUBA diving

Patient complains of ringing in the ears bilaterally

Patient complains of abnormal ear noises, which interfere with sleep and the ability to concentrate on his work

Patient complains that he feels a sense of tumbling, of falling backward associated with spinning of the room around him

She complains a sense of the ground rolling beneath her feet while walking in her office

Patient complains of persistent pain and discharge from the left ear for 2 months.

## PHYSICAL EXAMINATION OF EAR

Inspection reveals erythema and edema of the left ear canal skin with a purulent exudate.

Cerumen impaction is observed in the ear canal of left ear

Pinnae were normal to inspection bilaterally

Parotids are swollen bilaterally.

Postauricular pain and tenderness over the mastoid bone behind the right ear

Ears: Pinnae were normal on inspection, ear canals without abnormalities on inspection, tympanic membranes clear, no tenderness over the mastoid

# NOSE

**HISTORY**

Patient complains decrease in smell, nasal congestion, headache, sneezing, and scratchy nose.

She complains of discolored nasal discharge which is not responsive to decongestants

Mother reports that the child has the habit of nose picking and forceful nose blowing.

Patient complains of pain over the cheek, referring to the upper incisor and canine teeth.

He complains of a headache "in the middle of the head"

Patient complains of fever, chills, malaise, muscular aching, nasal stuffiness, substernal soreness, headache and nausea for the last 8 days.

**PHYSICAL EXAMINATION OF NOSE**

Nasal septum is deviated towards the right side

Inspection of the nasal mucosa shows black, necrotic eschar adherent to the inferior turbinate.

On inspection, the mucosa of the turbinates is violaceous

Purulent discharge through left nostril

Pain and tenderness over the maxillary sinus

Nose: Nasal septum showed no deviation; nasal turbinates not congested.

# MOUTH

**HISTORY**

Patient complains of decrease in taste, anorexia, weakness, irritability, mouth soreness, stomatitis, glossitis, and weight loss.

A white lesion is observed over the lateral tongue and floor of the mouth

She complains of burning and pain of the tongue.

Patient complains of tingling of the circumoral area, hands, and feet.

Patient complains of difficulty in chewing, inability to swallow or expel saliva, dysphagia and regurgitation of fluids through the nose

**PHYSICAL EXAMINATION OF MOUTH**

Fissures at the sides of the mouth (angular cheilitis)

Large amounts of thick tenacious saliva are present.

Small, round ulcerations surrounded by red halos are noticed on the buccal mucosa

Loss of papillae and red patches are noticed on the tongue—geographic tongue.

Mouth: Tongue on the midline, dentition good, no lesions, no vesicles, no oral thrush

# THROAT

## HISTORY

Patient complains of sore throat, increased pain with meals and a "hot potato" voice

Patient complains of high fever, chills, severe aching, headache, prostration, depression and sore throat

He complains of a rapidly developing sore throat, pain on swallowing and hoarseness of voice

Patient reports sudden onset of fever, sore throat, pain on swallowing, nausea, and malaise.

## PHYSICAL EXAMINATION OF THROAT

Creamy-white curd-like patches are seen overlying erythematous base.

Throat: No tonsillar enlargement, no erythema, no exudates, normal movement of the soft palate were noted, no deficit on phonation.

Inspection reveals a shaggy white-purple exudate over the tonsils

ENT:     Otoscopic examination reveals no abnormalities of external auditory canals and tympanic membranes. Inspection of nasal mucosa, septum and turbinates reveals erythema, exudate, inflammation, and pallor. Examination of nasopharynx reveals erythema. Inspection of tongue reveals normal color, good motility and midline position.

HEENT:   Congestion of the posterior pharyngeal wall. Pale nasal mucosa.

HEENT:   conjunctivae, pupillary reflexes, ENT were normal.

# NECK

## HISTORY

Patient complains of pain in the neck and radicular pain in the arm, exacerbated by head movement.

Patient presents with neck pain, restricted head movement, occipital headaches, radicular pain and weakness in the arms and legs

## PHYSICAL EXAMINATION OF NECK

Neck: supple without bruits, thyroid gland normal, cervical nodes negative, JVD pulse 4 cm above the sternal angle at head with bed elevation of 45 degrees

On inspection, a midline neck mass is observed just below the hyoid bone. The mass is moving with swallowing

Supple, thyroid gland normal, cervical nodes negative; no bruits detected.

Persistent cervical lymph nodes fixed to the skin are palpable.

Neck is supple. No goiter is appreciated.

Neck: supple, full ROM; no thyromegaly, no carotid bruits

Neck: Supple, trachea central, thyroid not enlarged, no jugular venous distention

# CARDIOVASCULAR SYSTEM

## HISTORY

### Dyspnea

Dyspnea is precipitated by walking roughly a half mile over a plane surface.

Dyspnea occurs abruptly around 20 minutes after going to bed and is relieved by sitting up or standing up.

### Chest pain

Chest pain occurs at rest and at night; occurs with exercise/emotion.

Chest pain associated with diaphoresis and left arm pain; not associated with nausea or vomiting; not relieved with antacids or meals.

Chest pain located retrosternally and radiating to the throat, lower jaw, shoulders, inner arms, upper abdomen and back

Patient complains of an instantaneous tearing pain of great intensity that is radiating to his back.

### Palpitations

Patient complains of rapid heart beat

42-year old male complaining of attacks of headache, palpitations and perspiration

### Elevated blood pressure

Patient reports that he had been hypertensive for the last 13 years

### Heart disease

Patient reports that he has mitral stenosis since 1987.

### Calf pain

Patient complains of pain in the calf muscles whenever he dorsiflexes his ankle

### Dizziness

Patient complains of dizziness and blurring of vision, whenever he adopts an upright position

### Syncope

Patient experiences loss of consciousness following a brief period of diaphoresis appr.3 times per day

# PHYSICAL EXAMINATION OF CARDIOVASCULAR SYSTEM

## JVD
JVD is normal
With bed elevation of 45 degrees, JVD pulse 4cm above the sternal angle.
S1, S2 normal; no added sounds or murmur.

## Pulse
Pulse is normal, small and slightly collapsing
Pulse is rapidly rising and collapsing

## PMI
Forceful, brisk PMI displaced significantly to left and down.
Powerful, heaving PMI to left and slightly below MCL.
PMI palpable on normal position.
PMI is non-displaced, palpable on normal position, no palpable heaves, pulses normal, no pedal edema
PMI fourth intercostal place within midclavicular line. S1, S2 regular rate and rhythm, no rubs, no murmurs
Palpable parasternal lift in the left parasternal area

## Thrill
Middiastolic thrill between lower left sternal border and PMI.

## Heart sounds
Loud snapping first mitral sound, opening snap following S2 along left sternal border.
Normal S1 and S2, prominent third heart sound
Normal S1, paradoxical splitting of S2, prominent S4

## Murmur
A loud, harsh systolic murmur in the left second and third interspaces parasternally
A loud, harsh holosystolic murmur is heard in the left third and fourth interspaces along the sternum.
Loud murmur in the right second intercostal space parasternally and also heard in carotids
Harsh, rough midsystolic murmur, begins after M1, ends before A2, accentuated with patient resting and leaning forward, with breath held in full expiration
Blowing, high-pitched, pansystolic murmur, loudest over PMI, transmitted to left axilla and left infrascapular area.
Low-pitched rumbling, middiastolic murmur, localized near apex.

**Concise Examples for Step-2 CS**
Normal rhythm, normal S1, S2, no murmurs, no thrills
Rhythm is irregular, normal S1 and S2 with no S3/S4 gallop, rubs or clicks
CVS: Normal S1, and S2 without murmurs, gallops, rubs, or clicks. Normal PMI
Regular rate and rhythm, normal S1, S2, no murmurs, no rubs, no gallops

# RESPIRATORY SYSTEM

## HISTORY
Patient complains of acute cough, which is described as productive. Severity of condition is moderate and worsening. Patient denies chest pain but complained of chest tightness intermittently and nocturnal cough. Patient indicates ambulation worsens condition.

She started having cough, fever, runny nose and sore throat, which have been getting worse over the period of time. Cough has been exhausting. She is bringing up yellowish expectoration. Associated with generalized weakness and palpitations. On asking, no palpitations.

### Dyspnea
Patient complains of dyspnea, hoarseness and a brassy cough
Patient complains of high fever, productive cough, rigors, dyspnea, occasional hemoptysis, and pleuritic chest pain.

### Cough
Persistent cough shortly after beginning the therapy with angiotensin converting enzyme inhibitors.
Patient complain of productive cough that followed upper respiratory tract infection

### Chest pain when breathing
Patient complains of chest pain and dyspnea on the affected side

### Hemoptysis
Patient has been coughing up blood since starting the inhalation of crack cocaine three months ago.

### Tuberculosis
Tuberculosis skin test was done in 2001 and found negative.

## PHYSICAL EXAMINATION OF RESPIRATORY SYSTEM
Breathing unlabored, rate 17/min
No deformities noted on inspection, normal inspiratory movements

No tenderness to palpation, tactile vocal fremitus within normal limits
No dullness to percussion
Normal breath sounds bilaterally, no wheezes, no rales, no rhonchi in any lung field

**Inspection**
Rate =14 breaths per minute
Rhythm = regular
Rhythm = rapid, shallow
Rhythm = rapid, large volume
Patient uses the accessory muscles of respiration, the intercostals and sternocleidomastoid muscles.
Digital clubbing is observed bilaterally.
Cyanosis of skin and mucous membranes
Inspiratory movements were normal

**Percussion**
Dull to percussion

**Palpation**
Mediastinum shifted to left side.
Axillae: both axillae were free of palpable nodes.

**Auscultation**
Lungs clear to auscultation
Auscultation of lungs reveals expiratory wheezes high-pitched and continuous bilateral.
Vesicular lung sounds are heard over the periphery of the lung
Bronchial lung sounds are heard over the suprasternal notch
Bronchial lung sounds are heard over the periphery of the lung.
BS were normal, no crackles, no wheezes.

**Concise form:**
Lungs clear to auscultation and percussion bilaterally; symmetric expansion; no dyspnea
Chest: there is bilateral good air entry. No crepitus. Bilateral expiratory rhonchi. Bilateral crackles

# ABDOMINAL SYSTEM

**HISTORY:**
**Dyspepsia**
Patient complains of epigastric discomfort, fullness, bloating, belching, and early satiety.
Patient complains of epigastric pain that is relieved by food or antacids.

Patient reports a gnawing, dull, aching, and 'hunger-like' pain in the epigastrium, often beginning 2 to 3 hours after taking a pill.

### Heartburn
Patient complains of a feeling of substernal burning, often radiating to the neck. The burning is exacerbated by meals, bending or recumbency.

### Anorexia
Patient reports anorexia, weakness, disturbed sleep, muscle cramps, impotence, loss of libido, sterility, and painfully enlarged breasts for the last two and a half months.

### Nausea and vomiting
Patient complains of vomiting of undigested food 1 hour after meals
Patient complains of severe abdominal pain, nausea, and vomiting immediately after meals.

### Hiccups
Patient complains of hiccups 5 to 10 minutes after drinking a carbonated beverage

### Constipation
Patient complains of hard, small, pellet-like stools on excessive straining during defecation

### Belching
Patient complains of eructation after meals and smoking
Patient reports that his belching after the ingestion of carbonated beverages is annoying to him and others around him

### Flatus
Patient complains of persistent, malodorous flatus after ingesting brown beans and broccoli

### Foul-smelling stools
Patient reports weight loss, flatulence, weakness, greasy and foul-smelling stools.

### Changes in consistency or color of stool
Patient complains of pruritis, malaise and light-colored stools
Patient reports weight loss, flatulence, large, loose to soft, pale-colored stools.
Patient complains of light-colored stools, dark urine, colicky pain in the right upper quadrant, weight loss, and jaundice.

### Diarrhea
Patient complains of increased frequency of bowel movements, 16 in the last 24 hours.
Patient reports watery, non-bloody diarrhea with periumbilical cramps, bloating and nausea.

## Melena
Patient states that he has been passing dark tarry stools for the last 6 days.

## Hematochezia
Patient complains of passage of sudden, painless, maroon blood during bowel movements.

## Hematemesis
Patient complains of vomiting brown 'coffee grounds' like material.
Patient stated she had vomited bright red blood twice in the past one week.
Patient presents with spontaneous emesis of bright red blood.

## Dysphagia
Patient complains of difficulties in swallowing foods, primarily for solid foods.
Patient reports coughing, choking, and regurgitation that occur immediately upon initiating swallowing.
Patient complains of the gradual onset of difficulties in swallowing for solid foods and of liquids and the need to throw his shoulders back in order to enhance esophageal emptying.

## Abdominal pain
Abdominal pain is intermittent, crampy, located in the lower abdominal pain and relieved by defecation
Patient reports sudden appearance of a severe, steady pain in the right hypochondrium after eating a large fatty meal.
Patient complains of abrupt onset of deep epigastric pain with radiation to the back.
Patient reports recurrent episodes of left upper quadrant pain with referral to the upper left lumbar region.

## Investigations
Colonoscopy was last performed in November 2002
Esophagogastroduodenoscopy was performed in January 99, which was normal.

## PHYSICAL EXAMINATION OF ABDOMEN

### INSPECTION
Globular abdomen on inspection
Abdomen is distended.
Six xanthomatous lesions around the left eyelid
Spider nevi are noticed on the upper half of the body.
Palmar erythema on the thenar and hypothenar eminences of left hand.

## AUSCULTATION

Normal abdominal bowel sounds

Normal abdominal bowel sounds but decreased on intensity and frequency.

Absent bowel sounds.

Soft, non-tender, non-distended to palpation, no hepatosplenomegaly, no rebound
tenderness, no CVA tenderness

Soft, nontender; Bowel sounds are present

## PERCUSSION

Abdomen tympanic to percussion in all 4 quadrants, dullness in the flanks, liver size
normal to percussion

Percussion: pain in the right lower quadrant on light percussion.

## PALPATION

Liver palpable, splenomegaly

No hepatosplenomegaly

On superficial palpation, the abdomen is tender mainly in the upper abdomen, without
guarding, rigidity, or rebound.

Tenderness in the right upper abdomen on superficial palpation

Pain in the left lower quadrant on deep palpation

Steady, severe pain and tenderness in the right hypochondrium, on superficial palpation.

On superficial palpation, there is tenderness in the right upper quadrant associated with
muscle guarding and rebound pain

Localized tenderness with guarding in the right lower quadrant

Rebound tenderness elicited

### Concise examples for Step-2 CS:

Bowel sounds present. Soft and nontender; No masses, hepatosplenomegaly, CVA
tenderness.

Abdomen: Soft, nontender, positive bowel sounds, negative for hepatosplenomegaly.

Abdomen: Soft, non tender, not distended, no organomegaly

# ENDOCRINE SYSTEM

## HISTORY

Patient complains of mild weight gain due to overeating.

Patient complains of losing weight despite increased appetite.

Patient complains of heat intolerance, attacks of nausea, abdominal pain, chest pain,
weakness, dyspnea, tremor, anxiety, weight loss, and visual disturbance.

Patient complains of sudden attacks of confusion, abnormal speech, loss of consciousness,
prolonged lethargy and dizziness.

This is a 59 year-old male with prostatic carcinoma taking diethylstilbestrol, complains of gynecomastia.

**PHYSICAL EXAMINATION OF ENDOCRINE SYSTEM**
Patient has plethoric, rounded and moon face along with prominent supraclavicular and dorsocervical fat pads.
Pigmentation of the upper lip, forehead, and malar eminences
Velvety brown pigmentation over the skin of the neck and axillae

# MUSCULOSKELETAL SYSTEM

**HISTORY**
Patient has a history of musculoskeletal low back pain secondary to lifting; fully evaluated in 1993, currently asymptomatic.
Patient complains of low back pain at night, unrelieved by rest or supine position
Patient complains of low back pain that worsens with rest and improves with activity.
Patient reports severe pain on the bottoms of their feet in the morning particularly with the first steps out of bed
Patient complains of bilateral lower back tenderness diffuse over the buttocks.
Patient complains of prominent stiffness in the morning, which subsides during the day
Patient complains of pain at the elbow with shaking hands or opening jars
Patient complains of difficulty in rising from a chair or climbing stairs
Patient complains of having trouble combing her hair, getting up out of a chair, and putting on a coat.
Patient presents with gait disturbance with gradual onset of unsteadiness in both legs that is precipitated by walking or prolonged standing and relieved by sitting.
Patient has a difficulty to arise from a sitting position and begin walking and a wide-based gait.

**PHYSICAL EXAMINATION OF MUSCULOSKELETAL SYSTEM**
**HEAD AND NECK**
Normal range of motion, flexion, extension, rotation and lateral movements were normal, no obvious deformities or signs of trauma, pain and tenderness to palpation of the posterior neck.
Cervical Foraminal Compression Test was positive bilaterally.

**SPINE**
No obvious deformities or signs of trauma
No spinous process or paraspinous tenderness
Normal range of motion—flexion, extension, rotation and lateral bending

## UPPER EXTREMITY

Shoulder: pain and tenderness over the right shoulder exacerbated by flexion, extension, and abduction movements, limited range of motion.

Elbow: normal flexion, extension, supination and pronation at the left elbow, limited range of motion were noted at right elbow on extension.

Wrist: normal radial and ulnar deviations of the hand at the wrist, pain and tenderness on flexion and extension movements.

Hand: no pain or tenderness on flexion and extension movements of the fingers of the both hands, no tenderness over the PIP and DIP joints of the both hands

Phalen's and Tinel's signs were positive on the Left hand and negative on the right hand.

## LOWER EXTREMITY

Hip: normal range of movements (flexion, extension, abduction, adduction, internal and external rotations) observed bilaterally, Straight Leg Raising Test was negative bilaterally, Trandelenburg test was negative bilaterally

Knee: normal flexion and extension, stability knee test was negative bilaterally, and McMurray's test was negative bilaterally Coarse crepitus is felt in the knee joint.

Joint effusion is present accompanied by a ballottable patella.

Tenderness was detected on knee flexion and extension movements.

McMurray's test is positive Range of motion in the knee is restricted Anterior drawer sign is positive Localized tenderness over the medial joint line

Ankle and Foot:

Flexion, extension, inversion and eversion were normal

No signs of trauma

Normal gait, reflexes were 2+ patellar, Achilles

## Back:

Pain and tenderness to palpation of the low back

Point tenderness over the 7th cervical vertebra.

## FOOT

Tenderness on the medial heel

Dorsalis pedis and posterior tibial are diminished on the left side.

## Concise examples for Step-2 CS:

Patient has ecchymosis involving foot ankle and lower leg. There is a small 4 cm swelling on anterior aspect of mid shin on left leg; normal gait; decreased range of motion noted in: left ankle flexion and eversion; pain with range of motion in: left ankle flexion and eversion; muscle strength: 5/5 in all major muscle groups.

Extremities: Negative for cyanosis, clubbing, edema

Extremities: No cyanosis, no clubbing, 1+ edema

Musculoskeletal system: Muscle strength full and symmetric, normal muscle tone without any atrophy or abnormal movements.

# NERVOUS SYSTEM

### HISTORY

Patient complains of temporary loss of consciousness preceded by pallor, nausea, malaise, sweating, accompanied by flaccidity.

Patient complains of headaches, which are worse on arising in the morning.

Patient reports falling to the ground accompanied by jerking of the body musculature.

Patient complains of seizures, impairment of external awareness, headache, nausea, disorientation, confusion, drowsiness, and soreness of the muscles.

Patient reports tremor, rigidity, slowness of voluntary movements and postural instability.

Patient complains of weakness and increased clumsiness on alternating sides of the body

Patient reports paralysis and loss of sensations in the face, the left arm, and the left leg.

Sudden and brief loss of vision

Patient complains of hallucinations, seizures, and impaired recent memory.

Patient recalls that the attack started with a sudden onset of impairment of consciousness, vomiting, severe headache and increased confusion.

### PHYSICAL EXAMINATION OF NERVOUS SYSTEM

Mental Status: alert, well oriented X 3, good concentration, MSE normal, speech normal rate, rhythm, tone, volume and content.

Cranial Nerves: 2-12 intact

Motor: strength of 5 of 5 all muscle groups

Sensory: sensory intact to pin, vibration, and proprioception

Reflexes: deep tendon reflexes 2+ responses symmetrically, plantar reflexes downgoing

Cerebellar: Romberg negative, finger to nose intact

Gait: normal

Tinel negative, Kernig negative, Brudzinski negative

Active, alert, and oriented X 3

Normal language and speech, able to follow commands well.

Cranial nerves 2-12 normal including optic, fundi, and visual fields.

Strength is 5/5 in the upper and lower extremities. Normal coordination, normal muscle tone, normal sensation.

Deep tendon reflexes are symmetric, +2

Plantar reflex response bilaterally, no calf tenderness

**Note:** Do not use non-specific terms like 'unremarkable' in patient note

| Practical Point for Patient Note on Reflexes: Normal Reflex = +2 |
| --- |

**Concise forms:**

Neuro: Awake, alert, oriented to time, place, and person, without facial deficit.

Neu: Higher functions are normal. CN are intact. There is no focal deficit.

CNS: essentially normal. Cranial nerves intact. No sensory or motor deficit

**Reflexes:**

Deep tendon reflexes were ¾

Delayed relaxation phase of reflexes is observed with all deep tendon reflexes.

Plantar reflexes downgoing

Patient has exaggerated deep tendon reflexes, absent superficial reflexes, and spastic paralysis

There are no focal neurological deficits. There is no pallor or icterus.

# PSYCHOLOGICAL STATUS

## HISTORY

Patient complains of intense fear of becoming fat and absence of menstrual cycles.

Patient reports uncontrolled ingestion of large quantities of food followed by self-induced vomiting, strict-dieting, vigorous exercise, and taking diuretics and cathartics

### Changes of mood

Patient reports mood elation with hyperactivity, increased irritability, flight of ideas, easy distractibility, little need for sleep, and over-involvement in life activities

Patient regrets that his previous life-style was characterized by excessive spending, exhibitionistic behavior, resignation from a good private-sector job, and a hasty marriage.

### Change in sleeping patterns

Patient complains of intermittent wakefulness during the night and early morning awakening.

Patient reports restless sleep, snoring, excessive daytime sleepiness, associated with headaches, memory impairment and depression.

Patient reports that his illness began with insomnia, apathy and irritability and progressed to memory loss, confusion, and hallucinations.

Patient complains of irritability, difficulty thinking, and confusion on awakening.

Patient has a history of marked withdrawal coupled with disturbed interpersonal relationships.

Patient has a history of polysurgery and alcohol dependence treated on multiple occasions with benzodiazepines.

## PSYCHIATRIC MENTAL STATUS EXAM

Remember the following mnemonic to write history from psychiatric patient

ACROSMA MAPS JITT

Expand and describe the components of the above mnemonic

Appearance: well groomed, appeared stated age

Consciousness: alert

Reasoning: good

Orientation: patient well oriented to time, place and person (A,O X 3)

Speech: fluent, normal rate, tone, and volume

Mood: depressed

Affect: sad

Memory: normal recent and remote memory

Attention: good

Perception: no illusions, no visual or auditory hallucinations

Suicidal Ideation: no suicidal ideation

Judgment: poor

Insight: fair

Thought processing: logical and goal-directed, no flight of ideas, no looseness of association, no tangentiality, no circumstantiality, no neologisms

Thought content: no suicidal ideation, no homicidal ideation, no delusions

## APPEARANCE

Appearance of being physically ill, irritable and less cooperative

Appears to be in distress, moderate unkempt blandness

## ATTITUDE

Patient is seductive and attention seeking

Patient is negativistic and quarrelsome

Patient is good mannered and cooperative

## CONSCIOUSNESS

Patient is able to spell WORLD backwards

Patient is not able to recall three objects at 5 minutes and recite the months of the year backwards

Patient is able to perform 'serial sevens test'

## REASONING

Reasoning is good

Reasoning is poor

## ORIENTATION
Alert, well oriented X 3
Oriented to place but not to time and person
Oriented to person and place but not to time

## SPEECH
Speech frequencies excellent
Patient's language is concrete and symbolic associated with rambling statements at times
    interspersed with mutism.
Patient's language is characterized by neologisms, echolalia, and verbigeration
Speech is normal rate and volume; fluent and coherent.

## MOOD
Mood is euthymic; affect is appropriate to material being discussed but he has a poor
    self-image.
Patient reports loss of interest and pleasure in usual activities, withdrawal from activities,
    feelings of guilt and worthlessness
Patient is dysphoric

## AFFECT
Flattened affect with occasional inappropriateness
Patient is angry and depressed
Affect: Sad
Affect: Appropriate
Affect: Congruent

## MEMORY
Patient failed to recall three objects at 5 minutes.
Patient is unable to spell 'WORLD backwards, repeat five digits and recite the months
    of the year backwards.

## ATTENTION
The patient interrupts his own sentences
Patient is less attentive, self-absorbed and easily distracting

## PERCEPTION

### Hallucinations
Patient complains of feeling blood flowing in blood vessels of his right forearm
Patient complains of a burning sensation on the left side of his brain whenever he thinks
    about his former girl-friend.

**Illusions**

Patient states that he had observed figures on his album changing in size constantly.

**Delusions**

Patient states that he had covered the ceiling of his dorm room with aluminum foil to counteract radar waves from Mars.

Patient states that he has been locking his home 24 hours a day as a countermeasure to prevent FBI agents entering his room.

**Depersonalization**

Patient complains of a feeling of being apart from the self.

**Distortion of body image**

Patient thinks his left hand has been decaying since his last birthday.

**SLEEP**

Patient complains of difficulty getting to sleep, staying sleep and early morning awakening.

Patient complains of excessive sleepiness, loss of muscle tone without loss of consciousness, disturbed nocturnal sleep, and vivid dream-like experiences during daytime naps

**JUDGMENT**

Judgment: good

Judgment: poor

**INSIGHT:** Insight is lacking, insight is superficial, insight is moderate, insight is profound

**THOUGHT PROCESS**

Patient's speech is characterized by flight of ideas, circumstantiality, and tangentiality.

Thought processes consists of looseness of association, neologisms and echolalia

**THOUGHT CONTENT**

Patient has fear of open places and public areas (Agoraphobia)

Patient has fears of annihilation since September 11, 2001.

Patient complains of constantly recurring thoughts of fears of exposure to germs

Patient has repetitive thoughts of engaging in violent activities against co-workers

Patient has obsessive thoughts about harming her 6 day-old baby boy.

**Physical Examination Model:**

PHYSICAL EXAM: GENERAL: The patient is pleasant, alert and oriented, in no acute distress. HEENT: Head is normocephalic, atraumatic. Extraocular muscles are intact.

Pupils equally round, reactive to light and accommodation. Oropharynx is clear with moist mucous membranes. Neck is supple with no lymphadenopathy and no JVD. HEART: Regular rate and rhythm. No murmurs, gallops or rubs. LUNGS: Clear to auscultation bilaterally. No rales, rhonchi or wheezing. ABDOMEN: Reveals mild left lower quadrant tenderness, but no guarding or rebound, nondistended and normal active bowel sounds. EXTREMITIES: Pulses +2 bilaterally, 2 to 3+ pitting edema bilateral lower extremities with the right being worse than the left. NEURO EXAM: Patient is alert and oriented x3. Cranial nerves II through XII grossly intact with no sensory deficits. Deep tendon reflexes are 2+. There is pain with range of motion of the right shoulder, otherwise the patient's strength is normal. MUSCULOSKELETAL:Pain with any movement of the right shoulder, otherwise full range of motion.

# 7

# FORMULATING THE DIFFERENTIAL DIAGNOSIS

Writing differential diagnosis involves comprising a list of possible conditions that are known to cause a particular clinical spectrum of signs or symptoms or both. Immediately following each patient encounter, the examinee will have ten minutes to complete a patient note. The physician should record pertinent medical history, physical examination findings, differential diagnosis and the necessary diagnostic studies.

As most cases in Step-2 CS are designed to present more than one diagnostic possibility, think about all possible diagnoses based on the information you obtain in the data gathering. Think about the possible differential diagnosis that reflect your findings in history taking and physical examination and list up to five of them from most likely to least likely. Your differential diagnosis should be derived from your patient findings, not some material you read in the textbooks. **Do not include non-relevant diagnoses just to fill the space.** There is no quick formula to frame an accurate differential diagnosis for a given clinical condition. Your basic clinical knowledge, history taking skills, physical examination techniques, and even communication skills all play a vital role in framing a relevant differential diagnosis of a disease.

**Golden rules to write a relevant differential diagnosis:**

1. *Think anatomically:* For example, in a patient with chest pain, imagine what are in the chest? Heart and Lungs. Then, think about conditions of heart and of lungs that produce chest pain. Now, you can think of some conditions like angina, MI, pleuritis etc. Similarly, in a female patient with RLQ abdominal pain, imagine what are located in RLQ? Appendix, Colon, Uterus, Ovary. Now, you can think of appendicitis, diverticulitis, Endometriosis, ovarian cyst etc according to the organ presented.
2. Make sure your list is derived from your history and physical findings.
3. Do not include non-relevant diagnoses just to fill space
4. Be specific, eg, do not write "abdominal disease" but rather 'appendicitis', 'peritonitis' etc.
5. Do not memorize the lists of differential diagnosis. This approach is more hazardous than helpful since you might be tempted to list down your differential

diagnosis from your memory instead of obtaining it from the clues you got from your history taking and physical examination. Remember each patient is unique. Develop a differential diagnosis for the patient's remarkable symptoms based on the pertinent positives and negatives of the history and physical examination, rather than quoting down from the pre-set memorized list of differential diagnosis of a particular disorder you read in a medical text book.

5. Also, use the knowledge of frequency and prevalence of disorders when writing the differential diagnosis.

6. Always consider the age of the patient when formulating the differential diagnosis because differential diagnoses of many symptoms varies with the age of the patient. For example, abdominal pain in a neonate is most commonly due to congenital intestinal atresia or stenosis, motility disorders etc; in infants and children due to gastroenteritis, colic, GE reflux, pyloric stenosis, appendicitis; in adolescents due to testicular or ovarian disorders; in adults due to neoplasms, pelvic inflammatory disease, ectopic pregnancy etc. In the same way, bone tumors are most likely primary in origin in patients younger than age 40 and metastatic in origin in patients older than 40. Similarly, Ewing's sarcoma is common in children and teens where as chondrosarcoma is common in adults older than 40 years.

7. Notice gender of the patient while considering the differential diagnosis. This will save you from writing ectopic pregnancy in a male patient complaining of abdominal pain, and writing BPH as the cause of difficulty urination in a female patient.

8. Remember your clinical knowledge, history, and physical examination will lead you to write the most relevant differential diagnosis, which in turn help you to form the diagnostic work-up.

**Rescue tip:** In the circumstances of nervousness, which is common in the time-constraining critical moments of Step-2 CS, use the mnemonic I MET PD, explained in full below, to derive your differential diagnosis.

It is the experience of many test takers to end up with blank minds when they are required to write out the differential diagnosis of a disorder. If you can not think of any related differential diagnosis from your memory, try to follow the following mnemonic and bring out any relevant causes from it.

**I MET PDs** ( I met Program Directors)
**Infections/Inflammations/Iatrogenic/Idiopathic causes**
**Metabolic causes**
**Endocrine/Electrolyte causes**
**Trauma/Tumor**
**Psychological causes/Pressure (hypertension)**
**Drug toxicity/Drug withdrawal**
**Sugar (Diabetes mellitus)**

# 70 MOST COMMON CASES FOR USMLE STEP-2 CLINICAL SKILLS

| Case Presentation | Differential Diagnosis | Diagnostic Workup |
|---|---|---|
| **Case #1**<br>40 year-old female complains of steady, severe pain in the right hypochondrium associated with fever, nausea and vomiting | Acute cholecystitis<br>Irritable bowel syndrome<br>Atypical appendicitis<br>Diverticulosis<br>Cholelithiasis | CBC<br>BMP<br>Urinalysis<br>Serum Amylase and lipase<br>X-ray abdomen<br>X-ray Chest |
| **Case #2**<br>30 year-old female complains of right lower quadrant abdominal tenderness, nausea, vomiting, and low-grade fever | Appendicitis<br>Diverticulitis<br>Crohn's disease<br>Pelvic inflammatory disease Ovarian torsion | CBC<br>BMP<br>CT Scan abdomen<br>Chest X-ray<br>Urinalysis |
| **Case #3**<br>60 year-old female complains of sudden onset of severe abdominal pain in the left upper quadrant associated with nausea and vomiting | Mesenteric Ischemia<br>Splenic Ischemia/Infarction<br>Left lower lobe Pneumonia<br>Pyelonephritis<br>Intestinal obstruction | CBC<br>BMP<br>X-ray abdomen<br>CT scan abdomen<br>Mesenteric arteriography |
| **Case #4**<br>67 year-old male complains of left lower abdominal pain associated with fever, nausea and vomiting | Diverticulitis<br>Ulcerative Colitis<br>Ovarian cyst<br>Pelvic Inflammatory Disease<br>Intestinal obstruction | CBC<br>BMP<br>Plain abdominal X-rays<br>CT Scan abdomen<br>Urinalysis |
| **Case #5**<br>Mother reports that her son got periorbital puffiness, weight gain, abdominal pain, presence of dark-colored urine and swollen feet | Nephrotic syndrome<br>Acute poststreptococcal glomerulonephritis<br>Hemolytic uremic syndrome<br>Henoch-Schoenlein purpura IgA nephropathy | CBC<br>Urinalysis<br>Urine culture<br>BUN/Creatinine<br>Renal sonography<br>Kidney biopsy |

| | | |
|---|---|---|
| **Case #6**<br>50 year-old female complains of recurrent episodes of epigastric pain associated with nausea, vomiting, constipation, flatulence and weight loss | Pancreatitis<br>Peptic ulcer<br>Gastric cancer<br>Celiac disease<br>Mesenteric vascular disease<br>Malignancy | CBC<br>BMP<br>Urinalysis & urine culture<br>Serum amylase & lipase<br>Stool for occult blood<br>Stool for ovum and parasites<br>X-ray abdomen<br>Chest x-ray<br>ECG<br>ERCP<br>CT abdomen |
| **Case #7**<br>63 year-old male complain of pain in the lumbosacral area which gets worse with prolonged standing and relieved by lying down | Herniated disc<br>Lumbar spondylosis<br>Spondylolisthesis<br>Compression fracture<br>Spinal cord tumor<br>Metastatic tumor | CBC<br>BMP<br>Urinalysis<br>ESR<br>X-ray of thoracolumbar spine |
| **Case #8**<br>55 year-old female complains of heaviness in chest increasing with exertion | Angina pectoris<br>Myocardial infarction<br>Myocarditis<br>Pericarditis<br>Esophagitis | CBC<br>BMP<br>ECG<br>Cardiac isoenzymes<br>Chest x-ray<br>Esophageal pH monitoring |
| **Case #9**<br>42 year-old male complains of fever, rigors, malaise, chest pain, wheezing and loss of appetite | Pneumonia<br>Upper respiratory tract infection<br>Chronic bronchitis<br>Congestive heart failure<br>COPD | CBC with differential count<br>BMP<br>Chest x-ray<br>Sputum smear & culture<br>Blood culture |
| **Case #10**<br>60 year-old female complains of difficulty falling asleep, weeps often as she contemplates her life, difficulty coping with family members | Depression<br>Adjustment disorder<br>Drug abuse<br>Posttraumatic Stress<br>Disorder Hypothyroidism | CBC<br>BMP<br>EEG<br>Drug screen<br>CT brain |

| | | |
|---|---|---|
| **Case #11**<br>70 year-old white male presents with two-day history of fever, crampy lower abdominal pain, and bloody diarrhea | Clostridium difficile colitis<br>Irritable bowel syndrome<br>Ulcerative colitis<br>Ischemic colitis<br>Giardiasis<br>Crohn's disease | CBC with differential<br>BMP<br>Stool for Clostridium difficile toxin<br>Stool for ova and parasites<br>Abdominal CT Scan |
| **Case #12**<br>65 year-old female complains of loose, watery stools daily for 2 weeks, abdominal pain, a general feeling of profound weakness | Celiac disease<br>Gastroenteritis<br>Inflammatory Bowel disease Irritable bowel syndrome Protein-losing enteropathy Malabsorption | CBC<br>Stool culture<br>Clostridium difficile toxin assay<br>ESR<br>Serum iron<br>CT Scan abdomen and pelvis |
| **Case #13**<br>65 year-old female complains of worsening dyspnea with walking one-third of a block, cough and wheezing | COPD Exacerbation<br>Bronchiectasis<br>Pulmonary fibrosis<br>Asthma<br>Congestive heart failure | CBC<br>BMP<br>Chest X-ray<br>Pulmonary Function Test<br>Chest CT Scan |
| **Case #14**<br>28 year-old male complains of suffering a new-onset generalized seizure while eating dinner | Epilepsy<br>AIDS encephalopathy<br>Hodgkin's disease<br>Conversion disorder<br>Hypoglycemia | CBC<br>BMP<br>EEG<br>CT Scan Head<br>Lumbar puncture for CSF exam |
| **Case #15**<br>50 year-old female complains of 1 to 2 bowel movements per week, stools are difficult to pass, hard and dry | Constipation<br>Intestinal obstruction<br>Abdominal hernia<br>Colon cancer<br>Ileus | CBC<br>TSH<br>Fecal occult blood<br>Abdominal CT Scan<br>Lower GI endoscopy |
| **Case #16**<br>75 year-old male comes in with increasing difficulty with urinating over the past two years, he gets up 5 times at night to urinate | Benign prostatic hypertrophy Prostatitis<br>Prostate cancer<br>Bladder stones<br>Bladder cancer<br>UTI | CBC<br>BUN and Creatinine<br>Urinalysis & urine culture<br>Prostate-Specific Antigen<br>Renal ultrasonography |

| | | |
|---|---|---|
| **Case #17**<br>24 year-old female complains of fever, general malaise, and fatigue | AIDS/HIV<br>Meningitis<br>Pneumonia<br>Pelvic inflammatory disease<br>UTI | CBC<br>Chest X-ray<br>Urinalysis and culture<br>Blood culture<br>HIV Antibody titer |
| **Case #18**<br>70 year-old female reports two-month history of fever, muscle weakness, night sweating, fatigue and arthralgia | Tuberculosis<br>Pneumonia<br>Malignancy<br>AIDS/HIV<br>Chronic Q fever | CBC<br>BMP<br>Sputum staining for Acid-fast bacilli<br>Chest X ray<br>Liver Function tests<br>Urinalysis and culture |
| **Case #19**<br>45 year-old female complains of palpitations for almost an hour, chest discomfort and mild shortness of breath | Panic attack<br>Atrial fibrillation/flutter<br>Ventricular tachycardia<br>Thyrotoxicosis<br>Pheochromocytoma<br>Digoxin toxicity | CBC<br>Serum electrolytes<br>Drug screen<br>TSH<br>ECG |
| **Case #20**<br>40 year-old woman complains of thick, foul-smelling vaginal discharge, mild back pain and abdominal pain | Trichomoniasis<br>Bacterial vaginosis<br>Candidiasis<br>Gonorrhea<br>Chlamydia | Vaginal pH<br>Whiff test<br>Light microscopy with KOH Urinalysis<br>CBC |
| **Case #21**<br>25 year-old female complains of a sore throat with swollen lymph nodes, fever, nausea and vomiting | Pharyngitis, viral<br>Pharyngitis, bacterial<br>Infectious mononucleosis<br>Hodgkin disease<br>Leukemia | CBC<br>BMP<br>Throat culture<br>Chest X-ray<br>Monospot test |
| **Case #22**<br>20 year-old female complains she is feeling extremely tired, she fainted while waiting in line in the cafeteria | Hypoglycemia<br>Hypotension<br>Aortic stenosis<br>Heart block<br>Sinus bradycardia<br>Sick sinus syndrome | Serum glucose<br>Serum electrolytes<br>CXR<br>ECG<br>Echocardiogram |

| Case #23 | | |
|---|---|---|
| 60 year-old male complains of shoulder pain, which is progressively getting worse for the last 3 years, pain increases with shoulder motion | Osteoarthritis<br>Rotator cuff injury<br>Shoulder subluxation<br>Acromioclavicular joint disease Glenohumeral arthritis<br>Gout arthritis | CBC<br>ESR<br>X-ray shoulder<br>MRI shoulder<br>EMG |
| **Case #24** | | |
| 14 year-old girl complains of amenorrhea, mild abdominal pain and irritability | Pregnancy<br>Imperforate hymen<br>Turner's syndrome<br>Polycystic Ovarian<br>Syndrome Hypopituitarism | TSH<br>HCG<br>Prolactin<br>FSH, LH<br>DHEAS<br>BUN Creatinine |
| **Case #25** | | |
| 70 year-old male complains of restlessness, agitation, mumbles incessantly and occasionally bursts into laughter | Delirium<br>Substance intoxication<br>Hypoglycemia<br>Depression<br>Psychosis | CBC<br>BUN and Creatinine<br>Urinalysis and urine culture<br>Liver function tests<br>Arterial blood gases<br>Drug screen<br>Liver function tests<br>Chest radiograph<br>Non-contrast-enhanced head CT |
| **Case #26** | | |
| 55 year-old man complains of difficulty swallowing, initially to solids and then liquids, resulting in mid-epigastric burning sensation and 20—pound weight loss | Achalasia<br>Primary esophageal tumor<br>Metastatic esophageal tumor Diffuse esophageal spasm Scleroderma esophagus | CBC<br>BMP<br>Chest radiography<br>Esophageal manometry<br>Barium esophagography |
| **Case #27** | | |
| 20 year-old male complains of painful enlargement of testicles, fever, increased urination and constipation | Epididymitis<br>Urethritis<br>Cystitis<br>Testicular tumor<br>Testicular torsion | CBC<br>Urinalysis & culture<br>Gram staining of urethral smear<br>BUN and creatinine<br>Scrotal ultrasound |

| | | |
|---|---|---|
| **Case #28**<br>60 year-old female complains of urinary incontinence with dull, intermittent lower abdominal pain | Urge incontinence<br>Stress incontinence<br>Overflow incontinence<br>Pelvic floor dysfunction<br>Urinary tract infection | Urinalysis<br>Cotton swab test (Q-tip)<br>Urodynamic study<br>Urinary cough stress test<br>Cystourethroscopy |
| **Case #29**<br>20 year-old female complains of extreme thirst that she wakes up several times during the night, frequent urination, fatigue and a 12 kg weight loss in the preceding 6 weeks | Diabetes mellitus<br>Nephrogenic Diabetes Insipidus, Central Diabetes Insipidus,<br>Craniophyringioma,<br>Psychogenic polydipsia | Serum glucose, serum Electrolytes, urine specific Gravity, urine sodium, serum<br>ADH level,<br>Pituitary MRI |
| **Case #30**<br>40 year-old man presented with low-grade fever, progressive pain in the genital region and urethral discharge | Urinary tract infection<br>Chlamydia<br>Gonorrhea<br>Prostatitis<br>Orchitis | CBC<br>Gram stain urethral smear<br>Urinalysis<br>Urine culture<br>HIV Testing |
| **Case #31**<br>75 year-old complains of difficulty speaking and right sided partial paralysis, which developed suddenly and continued for 30 minutes | Stroke, hemorrhagic<br>Stroke, Ischemic<br>Epidural hematoma<br>Elder abuse<br>Subarachnoid hemorrhage<br>Subdural hematoma | CBC<br>PT, aPTT, INR<br>Head CT Scan<br>MRI Brain<br>Lumbar puncture |
| **Case #32**<br>Weight loss<br>40 year-old female complains of intermittent abdominal pain and a 25 pound weight loss, diarrhea | Cholangitis<br>Cholecystitis<br>Diverticulitis<br>Mesenteric ischemia<br>Pancreatitis<br>Celiac sprue | CBC<br>AST&ALT<br>BUN & Creatinine<br>Amylase & Lipase<br>Ultrasound abdomen<br>ERCP |
| **Case #33**<br>60 year-old female complains of blurred vision and fatigue | Cataract<br>Glaucoma<br>Refractive error<br>Chorioretinitis<br>Optic atrophy<br>Papilledema | Slit lamp evaluation<br>Tonometry<br>Visual acuity evaluation<br>Visual fields<br>CT Scan head<br>CBC |

| | | |
|---|---|---|
| **Case #34**<br>60 year-old male complains of gradually progressive clumsiness and tremor of his right hand | Parkinson's disease<br>Familial tremor<br>Wilson's disease<br>Hyperthyroidism<br>Anxiety<br>Alcoholism<br>Caffeine intoxication | Drug screen<br>Alcohol screen<br>Serum copper<br>CT scan brain<br>EMG |
| **Case #35**<br>78 year-old male complains of tiredness, fatigue and hearing loss | Wax<br>Foreign body in the ears<br>Otosclerosis<br>Sensorineural deafness<br>Otitis media<br>Cholesteatoma<br>Acoustic neuroma | Audiometry<br>Caloric testing<br>Electronystagmography<br>Tympanography<br>X-rays of the mastoids<br>MRI brain |
| **Case #36**<br>60 year-old male complains that he snores and excessively sleepy all the time, wife sleeps in a different room | Obstructive sleep apnea<br>Narcolepsy<br>Hypothyroidism<br>COPD<br>Depression | CBC<br>TSH<br>Arterial Blood Gases<br>Lateral cephalometry<br>CT Scan<br>MRI |
| **Case #37**<br>60 year-old female complains of right knee pain, her pain limits her abilities to help her husband with routine tasks around their home | Osteoarthritis Knee<br>Traumatic arthritis<br>Infectious arthritis<br>Gout<br>Pseudogout | X-ray knee<br>Synovial fluid analysis<br>CBC<br>ESR<br>Blood culture |
| **Case #38**<br>25 year-old female complains of itching of perianal skin and pain with defecation | Enterobius vermicularis<br>Anal fistula<br>Anal fissure<br>Hemorrhoids<br>Genital warts<br>Seborrheic dermatitis | CBC cellophane tape<br>Scrapings of perianal skin<br>Transrectal ultrasound<br>Biopsy of perianal skin |

| | | |
|---|---|---|
| **Case #39**<br>30 year-old female complains of losing hair for the last 6 months, feeling tired and loss of appetite | Alopecia areata<br>Myxedema<br>hyperthyroidism<br>Malignancy<br>Tinea capitis<br>Seborrheic dermatitis | CBC<br>TSH<br>Serum iron and ferritin<br>Smear & culture of scrapings<br>Skin biopsy |
| **Case #40**<br>80 year-old female complains of rectal bleeding, dizziness, and unsteady gait | Hemorrhoids<br>Diverticulitis<br>Angiodysplasia<br>Carcinoma of colon<br>Ulcerative colitis<br>Crohn's disease<br>Ischemic colitis | CBC<br>Stool culture for ova and parasites<br>Serum electrolytes<br>Anoscopy<br>Barium enema<br>Radionuclide scan |
| **Case #41**<br>25 year-old female complains of decreased appetite, decreased sleep, lack of interest in her usual household activities, and reports that her heart is 'already absent' and her brain is 'shut off by aliens' | Major depression<br>Schizophrenia<br>Schizoaffective disorder<br>Bipolar disorder<br>Paranoid personality disorder<br>HIV encephalopathy | CBC<br>TSH<br>Urine toxicology screen<br>Liver function tests<br>HIV test<br>CT of brain |
| **Case #42**<br>22 year-old male presents with 3 days of nausea, vomiting, malaise, headache and imbalance | Viral gastroenteritis<br>Food poisoning<br>Hepatitis A or B<br>HIV<br>Meningitis<br>Diabetic ketoacidosis | CBC<br>BMP<br>Stool culture<br>HIV test<br>Serum electrolytes<br>CSF analysis |
| **Case #43**<br>36 year-old male complains of waking up in the middle of the night with a diffuse headache and a sensation of spinning when lying still with his eyes closed | Hypoglycemia<br>Hypovolemia<br>Hypoxia<br>Ménière disease<br>Benign Positional Vertigo<br>Vestibular neuronitis<br>Subclavian steal syndrome | CBC<br>BMP<br>Audiogram<br>Caloric test<br>MRI brain<br>EEG |

| | | |
|---|---|---|
| **Case #44**<br>80 year-old female complains of drowsiness, vomiting and severe sudden headache | Subarachnoid hemorrhage<br>Subdural hematoma<br>Acute stroke<br>Meningitis<br>Cerebral venous thrombosis, Migraine | CBC<br>BMP<br>PT,aPTT<br>CT head<br>Lumbar puncture<br>Cerebral angiography |
| **Case #45**<br>50 year-old female complains of progressive shortness of breath, a productive cough with blood-tinged sputum | Lung carcinoma<br>Bronchiectasis<br>Pulmonary embolism<br>Pneumonia<br>Tuberculosis | CBC<br>CMP<br>PT,INR,aPTT<br>Sputum smear,culture<br>Chest X-ray<br>Sputum for AFB |
| **Case #46**<br>65 year-old woman complains of urge to void that comes urgently, and she 'can't make it to the bathroom in time' | Urge incontinence<br>Urinary tract infection<br>Stress incontinence<br>Overflow incontinence<br>Urethral obstruction | CBC<br>Urinalysis & culture<br>BMP<br>Intravenous pyelogram<br>Voiding cystogram<br>Cystoscopy |
| **Case #47**<br>25 year-old female complains of acute lower abdominal pain and pain during intercourse | Pelvic inflammatory disease Endometriosis<br>Ectopic pregnancy<br>Urinary tract infection<br>Torsion of ovarian cyst | CBC<br>Pregnancy test<br>Urinalysis & culture<br>Vaginal smear & culture<br>Pap smear<br>Pelvic ultrasound |
| **Case # 48**<br>36 year-old male complains of weakness, fatigue and heartburn | Reflux esophagitis<br>Gastritis<br>Peptic ulcer<br>Cholecystitis<br>Cholelithiasis<br>Coronary insufficiency | CBC<br>Esophagoscopy<br>Gastroscopy<br>Gall bladder ultrasound<br>Esophagus pH |
| **Case # 49**<br>75 year-old male complains of difficulties with sleep initiation, staying asleep as he is unable to 'shut off his mind' | Sleep apnea<br>Chronic anxiety<br>Depression<br>Alcohol intoxication<br>Drug intoxication | CBC<br>Drug screen<br>TSH<br>Serum alcohol level<br>CT scan brain |

| | | |
|---|---|---|
| **Case # 50**<br>75 year-old female reports short-term memory loss of 2 years duration, loss of interest in daily activities, decline in attention and concentration | Alzheimer disease<br>Dementia with Lewy bodies Depression<br>Hypothyroidism<br>Vitamin B12 deficiency | CBC<br>TSH<br>Vitamin B12 level<br>Brain MRI<br>SPECT |
| **Case # 51**<br>14 year-old male complains of ear discharge, progressive restlessness, fever and cough | Otitis media<br>Foreign body in ear<br>Mastoiditis<br>Otitis externa<br>Labyrinthitis | CBC<br>BMP<br>X-rays of the mastoid<br>Tympanometry<br>Blood cultures<br>Nasopharyngoscopy |
| **Case # 52**<br>40 year-old male complains of hoarseness of voice, his voice fatigues near the end of the day and he starts to cough | Laryngitis<br>Laryngotracheobronchitis<br>Laryngeal malignancy<br>GERD<br>Bronchitis | CBC<br>Laryngoscopy<br>24-hour pH probe |
| **Case # 53**<br>Mother reports that her 3 month-old boy is currently at his birthweight of 3.9 mg, poor feeding, nonbilious emesis, and she fears that her baby is not growing well | Child abuse<br>Fetal alcohol syndrome<br>Food allergy<br>Pancreatic insufficiency<br>Cystic fibrosis | CBC urinalysis<br>Electrolytes, creatinine,<br>BUN Prealbumin<br>HIV testing<br>Serum amylase and lipase<br>sweat chloride test |
| **Case # 54**<br>66 year-old male with history of diabetes complains of chronic non-healing ulcers on his right foot | Diabetic foot ulcer<br>Atherosclerosis<br>Chronic venous insufficiency<br>Malignant melanoma<br>Squamous cell carcinoma | CBC<br>Serum glucose<br>Glycohemoglobin<br>Ankle-brachial blood pressure index<br>Duplex scanning<br>Biopsy of ulcer |

| | | |
|---|---|---|
| **Case # 55**<br>45 year-old male complains of failure to achieve erection, fatigue, malaise, and low back pain | Peripheral arterial occlusive disease<br>Prostitis<br>Prostate cancer<br>Depression<br>Hyperpituitarism | Serum testosterone<br>LH & Prolactin<br>Urinalysis<br>Total cholesterol,HDL,LDL<br>Transrectal ultrasonography |
| **Case # 56**<br>45 year-old male complains of indigestion, abdominal bloating, and constipation | Gastric ulcer<br>Esophagitis<br>Duodenal ulcer<br>Pancreatitis<br>Intestinal obstruction | CBC<br>Endoscopy<br>TSH<br>Esophageal pH monitoring<br>Stool for occult ovum & parasites |
| **Case # 57**<br>60 year-old male complains of a sensation of tingling, pricking, or numbness of both lower limbs followed by difficulty controlling voluntary movements and widebased gait | Normal pressure hydrocephalus<br>Vitamin B12 deficiency<br>Folate deficiency<br>Alcoholism<br>Neurosyphilis | CBC<br>Serum cobalamin level<br>Serum folate level<br>Serum alcohol level<br>Brain MRI |
| **Case # 58**<br>45 year-old male complains of abdominal pain and melena | Upper GI bleed<br>Lower GI bleed<br>Gastric ulcer<br>Duodenal ulcer<br>Malignancy | CBC<br>PT,aPTT,INR<br>Stool for occult blood<br>Stool for ovum & parasites<br>Endoscopy |
| **Case # 59**<br>17 year-old female complains of fatigue, dizziness, loss of appetite, extreme weight loss, dry skin and hair, irritability and social withdrawal | Anorexia nervosa<br>Depression<br>Anxiety Disorder<br>Alcohol and Substance abuse Hyperthyroidism | CBC<br>Serum electrolytes<br>Chest X-ray<br>TSH<br>AST,ALT,Albumin level |

| | | |
|---|---|---|
| **Case # 60**<br>32 year-old complains of not being able to get pregnant after one year of trying | Pelvic inflammatory disease<br>Stenosis of cervix<br>Turner's syndrome<br>Hypothyroidism<br>Retroverted Uterus | CBC<br>Urinalysis & culture<br>Cervical smear and culture<br>TSH<br>Hysterosalpingogram<br>Pelvic ultrasound |
| **Case # 61**<br>40 year-old female complains of flank pain, fever, shaking chills, and pain with urination | Pyelonephritis<br>Appendicitis<br>Cholecystitis<br>Diverticulitis<br>Lower lobe pneumonia | CBC with differential<br>Urinalysis<br>Urine culture<br>Chest X-ray<br>Renal ultrasound |
| **Case # 62**<br>35 year-old female complains of dryness, pain with sexual intercourse associated with loss of interest in sexual activities | Atrophic vulvovaginitis<br>Pelvic inflammatory disease Endometriosis<br>Lichen sclerosus<br>Vaginismus | CBC<br>Urinalysis & culture<br>Vaginal smear and Culture<br>Pelvic ultrasound<br>Vaginal biopsy |
| **Case # 63**<br>25 year-old female complains of a 3 cm round, nontender mass in her right breast | Fibroadenoma<br>Cystadenoma<br>Breat abscess<br>Chronic mastitis<br>Breat carcinoma | CBC<br>Mammography<br>Ultrasonography<br>Fine needle aspiration<br>Biopsy |
| **Case # 64**<br>40 year-old female complains of fatigue, dry skin, forgetfullness, muscle weakness | Anemia<br>Depression<br>Fibromyalgia<br>Diabetes mellitus<br>Hypothyroidism | CBC<br>CMP<br>TSH<br>HIV testing<br>Urinalysis |
| **Case # 65**<br>30 year-old male complains of pain in the back of his neck, gets worse with neck motions | Cervical strain or sprains<br>Herniated nucleus pulposus<br>Osteoarthritis<br>Ankylosing spondylitis<br>Rheumatoid arthritis<br>Fibromyalgia<br>Osteomyelitis<br>Polymyalgia rheumatica<br>Compression fracture | Serum calcium<br>ESR<br>X-rays of cervical spine<br>MRI cervical cord<br>Electromyography |

| | | |
|---|---|---|
| **Case # 66**<br>60 year-old male complains of urine output of less than 100 ml per day, malaise, vomiting, lower abdominal pain | Acute renal failure<br>Renal calculi<br>Urinary obstruction<br>Urinary tract infection<br>Dehydration | CBC<br>CMP,CPK<br>Urine output measurement<br>Urinalysis & culture<br>Fractional Excretion of Sodium |
| **Case # 67**<br>73 year-old female complains of right hip pain that worsens with activity and weightbearing, she also started to limp to avoid the pain | Osteoarthritis<br>Hip fracture<br>Avascular necrosis<br>Bone metastases<br>Osteomyelitis | CBC,ESR<br>Serum protein electrophoresis<br>X-ray lumbosacral spine & hip<br>Bone scan<br>MRI lumbar spine & hip |
| **Case # 68**<br>35 year-old male complains of heart burn, difficulty eating and vomit that looks like coffee grounds | Esophagitis<br>Esophageal varices<br>Gastric cancer<br>Gastric ulcer<br>Boerhaave syndrome | CBC with differential<br>CMP<br>PT,aPTT,INR<br>Chest X-ray<br>Endoscopy |
| **Case # 69**<br>14 year-old male complains of increased breast size, nipple discharge, decreased libido and strength | Gynecomastia<br>Hypogonadism<br>Lipoma<br>Lymphangioma<br>Breast Cancer<br>Dermoid Cyst | CBC<br>Serum testosterone<br>LH estradiol<br>TSH |
| **Case # 70**<br>10 year-old male complains of bleeding from the nostrils and nausea | Trauma<br>Foreign body in nose<br>Hemophilia A<br>Hemophilia B<br>Sinusitis | CBC<br>Platelet count<br>Bleeding time<br>PT/INR<br>CT scan sinuses |

# 8

# ORDERING THE DIAGNOSTIC WORK UP

Your diagnostic work up is the list of diagnostic tests you are going to order to narrow down your differential diagnosis to one definitive diagnosis. Thus your diagnostic work up should flow from the differential diagnosis you made after your patient encounter. If you think rectal, pelvic, genitourinary, female breast, or corneal reflex examinations should be done as part of the evaluation for that specific patient, you may include them in your diagnostic workup plan on the patient note.**Remember that your diagnostic work up should be based on your history taking and physical examination. This fact should be considered for every test you order.**

Helpful guidelines to write the patient note:

1.  Carefully select the investigations you are going to order. Do not order expensive, non-indicated diagnostic tests in the place of inexpensive, indicated diagnostic tests.
2.  Do not indicate tests just to fill the spaces
3.  Avoid unnecessary investigations. You must be able to justify the need for each diagnostic investigation you are going to order. Remember no diagnostic test is 'routine'.
4.  Prefer reasonable non-invasive, low risk alternative to an invasive, high risk investigation.
5.  Discuss with the patient the potential complications and risks of the investigations you are going to order, especially if the investigations are invasive.
6.  Avoid diagnostic work up plans that could result in harm.
7.  Write only first line and specific tests.
8.  Do not include treatment plans
9.  Do not include hospitalization, consultation, or referrals
10. Order specific tests rather than a group of 'studies' or 'series. For example, do not order "SMA-20", "Chemistry panel", or "Liver profile", but rather, the specific component tests you are interested in, e.g., "BUN, glucose, Na, K."

Order T4, TSH instead of "thyroid studies" or "thyroid panel"
Order AST, ALT, AKA instead of "liver profile"
Order BUN, Creatinine instead of "renal studies"

11. List up to five diagnostic tests from the most relevant to the less relevant.
12. If you are without a clue, think about the system involved in the presenting case, and imagine the most important studies you normally perform to visualize that system.

   For example, if the presenting complaint is cough with expectoration, the system involved is the respiratory system and the most important diagnostic test is Chest X-ray.
   If the chief complaint is stroke, the system involved is the nervous system and the most important diagnostic test is CT Scan.
   If the chief complaint is pain with urination, the system involved is the urinary tract and the most important diagnostic test is Urinalysis and culture
   You can use CBC with differential for almost every case

13. Remember the sex of the patient while writing down the labs. This will help you avoid ordering pregnancy test in a male patient or PSA in a female patient.

# DIAGNOSTIC TESTS AND THEIR APPLICATION
# CARDIOVASCULAR SYSTEM

**Angiography:** An imaging technique in which radiocontrast is injected into the cardiac arteries to identify obstructions or vascular defects. It is used to detect abnormalities such as aneurysms in the blood vessels and the organs they serve. It can be used for both diagnostic and therapeutic radiography of the heart and blood vessels.

*Indications:*
   1. to study coronary arteries for degenerative narrowing or blockage
   2. to assess the size of arteries for the formation of aneurysms
   3. to assess congenital malformations of arteries

**Apolipoproteins**: Apolipoproteins are the major protein components of blood fats, of which LDL and HDL are examples. The ration of LDL and HDL is very useful in identifying at-risk persons for coronary artery disease.

*Indications:* Persons at risk for atherosclerosis and coronary artery disease.

**Aspartate aminotransferase(AST):** Aspartate aminotransferase is an enzyme found primarily in heart muscle and liver. High levels of AST are found following acute MI and serum levels increase 10 times or more and remain high in liver disease.

*Indications:* acute myocardial infarction, severe angina, hepatitis, cancer of liver, alcoholism, acute pancreatitis, cerebral infarction, trauma, diabetic ketoacidosis, chronic liver disease

**Cardiac catheterization:** Cardiac catheterization aids in the visualization of the heart and the coronary arteries. In cardiac catheterization, a long, slim hollow catheter is threaded into an artery or vein in the upper groin or arm. This catheter is gently threaded through the vessel to the heart and a radiographic dye is injected. This dye outlines the heart, vessels, and pressure gradients across the valves.

*Indications:*
1. to diagnose coronary artery disease with specific information about atherosclerotic arteries.
2. To diagnose congenital abnormalities, intracardiac tumors, ventricular mural thrombi, septal defects, aneurysms, and valvular defects.
3. To diagnose atypical chest pain, complication of Myocardial infarction, aortic dissection, coronary artery surgery or angioplasty
4. To assess valvular function

**Cardiac isoenzymes:** CK-MB and LDH1 and LDH2
Cardiac isoenzymes are those enzymes that are specifically released from the cardiac muscle. These enzymes are released when tissue cells are damaged and can be detected and measured in the serum. CK-MB, LDH 1 and LDH 2, Troponin are cardiac-specific isoenzymes.

*Indications:*
**CK-MB:** to diagnose acute myocardial infarction
**LDH 1 and LDH 2, Troponin**: to diagnose myocardial infarction

**NOTE:** In Step-2 CS, write specifically as CK-MB, Troponin instead of writing "cardiac isoenzymes".

**Carotid doppler:** a carotid Doppler examination is a noninvasive procedure that examines the arteries supplying the brain.

*Indications:*
1. to evaluate suspected atherosclerotic clinical manifestations (e.g., headache, dizziness, paresthesia, speech difficulties, and visual disturbances).
2. To diagnose carotid plaque, stenosis, occlusion, dissection, aneurysm, and carotid body tumor

**Cholesterol:** Because increased cholesterol levels have been associated with atherosclerosis, coronary artery disease, and an increased risk of death due to heart attacks, cholesterol is commonly measured and included in most routine chemistry panels.

*Indications:* Cholesterol testing is most frequently done as a screening tool for atherosclerotic coronary disease and is also a component of thyroid and liver function studies

**Doppler ultrasonography:** Doppler Ultrasonography is a noninvasive test that uses ultrasound waves to study blood flow and identify occlusions of the veins or arteries. Ultrasound diagnosis differs from radiological diagnosis in that there is no ionizing radiation involved.

*Indications:* to diagnose arterial aneurysms, small or large vessel occlusions, Raynaud's phenomena, chronic venous insufficiency, aortic stenosis, embolic arterial occlusive disease, venous occlusions, and varicose veins.

**Electrocardiography:** Electrocardiography is a noninvasive testing of the electrical output of the heart. This test uses all 12 electrode leads and is able to evaluate 360° of vectors that reflect the electrical functioning of the heart.

*Indications:* evaluates and monitors angina pectoris, anxiety, dysrhythmias, bradycardia, carbon monoxide poisoning, chest pain, CHF, endocarditis, MI, panic disorder, pulmonic stenosis, pacemaker function, pericarditis, respiratory distress, ventricular hypertrophy, and a wide variety of cardiac disorders.

**Holter monitoring:** The Holter monitor involves the use of a small portable ECG monitor, which the client wears. This monitor enables the continuous recording of the client's cardiac electrical activity on tape.

*Indications:* evaluates electrical activity in the client who is experiencing symptoms suggestive of a possible cardiac rhythm disturbance.

**Pericardiocentesis:** Pericardiocentesis is the removal of fluid from the pericardial sac.

*Indications:* to diagnose viral pericarditis, hemorrhagic pericarditis, Dressler's syndrome, to rule out carcinoma, tuberculosis and fungal infections.

**Stress exercise:** The stress exercise test measures cardiac efficiency while the heart is being stressed through exercise. It records the patient's heart beats while he or she is walking on a treadmill.

*Indications:*
1. to diagnose a possible cardiac cause of symptoms such as chest pain, shortness of breath or lightheadedness
2. to diagnose coronary artery disease
3. to check the effectiveness of procedures done to improve coronary artery circulation in patients with coronary artery disease

**Transesophageal echocardiogram:** A transesophageal echocardiogram involves the passage of an ultrasound transducer into the esophagus. The ultrasound produces high-frequency sound waves to induce vibrations to visualize images of heart size, shape, volume, left-ventricular wall motion, valve function, and possible source of emboli.

*Indications:*
1. to detect any irregularity in heart size, wall function, and valve function
2. diagnoses cardiac tumors
3. detects mitral valve regurgitation
4. detects congenital heart disorders of the adult
5. determines aortic dissection site and extent

**Cardiac Scans**

Cardiac scan involves intravenous administration of the isotope followed by a scan or series of scans. There are four major types of cardiac scans:

1. Technetium pyrophosphate scan: This scan can confirm a recent myocardial infarction and determine the extent and exact location of damage to the heart muscle.
2. Thallium imaging: In this scan, the thallium isotope accumulates in normal heart muscle, rather than infarcted regions, and produces 'cold spots' on the screen.
3. MUGA scan: MUGA scan evaluates the motion of the heart wall to detect abnormalities such as valve problems, aneurysms, coronary artery disease or heart attack.
4. PET Scan: PET Scan uses positron-emitting isotopes to assess the viability of and blood flow to the cardiac muscle. It provides more information about the cardiac muscle than other imaging techniques.

*Indications:*
1. to diagnose coronary artery disease
2. to stratify the risk of stable angina, unstable angina, and post-myocardial infarction

**Triglycerides:** Triglycerides are a combination of glycerol with different fatty acids. The test evaluates for atherosclerosis and thus the body's ability to metabolize fats.

*Indications:* Triglyceride testing is used in combination with cholesterol and fatty acid testing when clients have cardiovascular disturbances.

**Troponin T:** Troponin is an inhibitory protein found primarily in cardiac muscle. Troponin is released with relatively small amounts of cardiac injury in as early as 1-3 hr and will remain elevated for 2 weeks postinjury.

*Indications:* to detect Myocardial Infarction
To identify the severity of cardiac disorder

**Cold Stimulation Test**
Cold stimulation test measures temperature changes in the fingers after exposure to cold.
*Indications:*
To assess the patients with suspected vasospastic disorders
1. Raynauds syndrome
2. Rheumatoid arthritis
3. Scleroderma
4. Systemic Lupus Erythematosus

**Phlebography**
Phlebography aids in the x-ray visualization of the veins in the legs and feet.

*Indications:*
1. to diagnose deep venous thrombosis
2. to evaluate congenital abnormalities in the veins
3. to distinguish between blood clots and other obstructions such as tumors

# ENDOCRINE SYSTEM

**ACTH:** ACTH is a hormone secreted by the anterior pituitary gland that signals the adrenal gland to release steroids (cortisol, androgens, and aldosterone), critical to the normal functioning of the body. In patients with Cushing's syndrome, ACTH measurement is extremely important because ACTH levels help determine where the lesion is located.

*Indications:* to establish a diagnosis of Addison's disease, Cushing's syndrome, Pituitary adenomas and malignant tumors that produce ACTH and pituitary and hypothalamic disease.

**ACTH stimulation test:** With ACTH stimulation Test, elevated levels of cortisol are found when the adrenal glands are functioning normally, and decreased levels are found if adrenals are not functioning normally.

*Indications:*
1. to establish whether the adrenals are responding
2. tto help differentiate adrenal disease from pituitary or hypothalamus disease.

**ADH:** Antidiuretic hormone is released by the posterior pituitary in response to increased blood osmolality or decreased blood volume

*Indications:* to diagnose diabetes insipidus, SIADH, lung cancer etc.

**Calcitonin:** Calcitonin is a hormone produced and secreted by C cells of the thyroid gland. Its action is opposite to that of parathyroid hormone, in that calcitonin increases deposition of calcium and phosphate in bone and lowers the level of calcium in the blood. Patients with medullary thyroid cancer will excrete elevated levels of calcitonin.

*Indications:* To diagnose medullary thyroid cancer

**Calcium:** Calcium is the most abundant mineral in the body, of which over 90% is stored in the skeleton and the teeth. Serum calcium levels include both ionized and protein-bound calcium since they cannot be measured independently.

*Indications:*
1. To diagnose hyperparathyroidism, hypoparathyroidism, Paget's disease, Multiple myeloma, and Vitamin D toxicity or deficiency
2. To assist in diagnosis of acid-base imbalance, coagulation disorders, pathologic bone disorders, endocrine disorders, cardiac arrhythmia, muscle disorders

**Cortisol Tests:**
Cortisol stimulatory test uses an infusion of ACTH for confirmation of the diagnosis of hypofunction of the adrenal gland.

Cortisol suppression test uses dexamethasone for confirmation of the diagnosis of hyperfunction of the adrenal gland. This test is performed by administering dexamethasone to determine the effect on cortisol production. It is done as part of the diagnostic investigation for Cushing's syndrome. (Dexamethasone Suppression Test)

*Indications:*
1. to diagnose Cushing's Syndrome, Cushing's disease, and primary and secondary adrenal insufficiency
2. To distinguish between primary and secondary adrenal insufficiency

## Estrodiol
It is a steroid produced by the ovary and possesses estrogenic properties. It diminishes or stops during menopause.

*Indications:*
1. To evaluate female infertility, amenorrhea, menstrual irregularity, or sexual precocity in the child
2. To evaluate a feminizing condition in the male

## Estriol, pregnancy
It is found in the urine of women. It is an estrogenic hormone considered to be the metabolic product of estrone and estradiol.

*Indication:* to evaluate fetal well-being and placental function especially in the high-risk pregnancy

## Estrogen, total
Natural estrogens include estradiol, estrone, and their metabolic product, estriol.

*Indications:*
1. To evaluate ovarian function, predict ovulation
2. To evaluate excess or decreased estrogen conditions
3. To determine the cause of amenorrhea
4. To help diagnose a testicular tumor

## Follicle-Stimulating Hormone
FSH is hormone that regulates the growth and development of eggs and sperm. FSH test is a blood test in which blood is drawn from the patient and analyzed in a laboratory to diagnose or evaluate disorders involving the pituitary gland and reproductive system.

*Indications:*
1. to diagnose pituitary disorders

2. to determine if the menopause has begun to diagnose infertility in the female and testicular dysfunction in the male
3. to diagnose menstrual disorders such as anovulatory bleeding
4. to evaluate patients with anorexia nervosa

## Glucagon

Glucagon is a polypeptide hormone secreted by the alpha cells of the pancreas that increases the blood glucose level by stimulating the liver to change stored glycogen to glucose.

*Indications:*
To assess in suspected pancreatic tumors, chronic pancreatitis, familial hyperglucagonemia

## Glucose Tolerance Test

The glucose tolerance test determines the body's ability to metabolize glucose after administration of an oral carbohydrate challenge. An abnormal glucose tolerance test aids to confirm diabetes mellitus.

*Indications:* To diagnose Diabetes Mellitus

## Blood Glucose Test

Glucose is the end product of the carbohydrate digestion. In healthy people, normal blood glucose levels are maintained at about 70 to 110 mg/dl.

*Indications:*
1. To assess and manage patients with Diabetes Mellitus
2. To monitor other hyperglycemic patients, such as those patients on hyperalimentation or high-dose glucocorticoid therapy

## Urine Glucose Test

Urine glucose or urine sugar test is used to measure the amount of glucose in urine.

*Indications:*
1. to diagnose diabetes
2. to monitor adequacy of diabetic control
3. When capillary glucose monitoring is not possible, urinary glucose is measured to determine insulin and dietary requirements

## Glycosylated Hemoglobin(Hemoglobin A1)

It is Hemoglobin A that contains a glucose group linked to the terminal amino acid of the beta chains of the molecule. It is a good indicator of long-term glycemic control. It is not affected by recent changes in diet or medication, like fasting blood glucose. Diabetics who are poorly controlled will have a glycosylated hemoglobin value that is more than 12% of the total hemoglobin value

*Indications*
To assess diabetic control

## Growth Hormone
Growth hormone is secreted by the anterior pituitary,which regulates the cell division and protein synthesis necessary for normal growth. Tests for growth hormone include Somatotropin hormone test, Somatomedin C, Growth hormone suppression test, and Growth hormone stimulation test.

*Indications:*
1. to identify growth deficiencies such as delayed puberty and small stature
2. to diagnose gigantism or acromegaly
3. to assist in the diagnosis of pituitary tumors or tumors related to the hypothalamus

## Insulin
Insulin is a hormone secreted by the beta cells of the pancreas that controls the metabolism and cellular uptake of sugars, proteins, and fats.

*Indications:*
1. To assess for insulin producing tumors
2. To confirm suspected insulin-resistant states.

## Ketone bodies Test
Acetone, Acetoacetic acid, and beta-hydroxybutyric acid are called ketone bodies.

*Indications:*
1. To evaluate the patients with diabetes mellitus and to diagnose carbohydrate deprivation in urine
2. To distinguish between diabetic ketoacidosis and hyperosmolar coma in serum
3. To adjust insulin requirements in the diabetic and to monitor patients on low-carbohydrate diets in urine

## Parathyroid hormone, serum
It is a hormone produced by parathyroid gland that regulates calcium and phosphorus metabolism.

*Indications:*
1. To diagnose suspected parathyroid disorders

2. To differentiate between clinical diagnoses that result in calcium and phosphate abnormalities

**Progesterone, serum**
It is a steroid hormone obtained from the corpus luteum and placenta.

*Indications:*
1. To determine ovulation
2. To assess the function of the corpus luteum, particularly in cases of habitual abortion or infertility

**Radioactive Iodine Uptake (RAIU) or Iodine uptake test**
A test of thyroid function that measures the amount of orally ingested radioactive iodine that accumulates in the thyroid gland. It can be used to evaluate thyroid function, particularly when blood tests of thyroid function (for example, T3 and T4) have abnormal results.

*Indications:*
1. Hashimoto's thyroiditis
2. Hyperthyroidism
3. Hypothyroidism
4. Subacute thyroiditis

**Antithyroid microsomal antibody** (or thyroid antimicrosomal antibody) **test**
It is a test used to measure antithyroid microsomal antibodies in the blood.

*Indications:*
1. to confirm the cause of thyroid problems or other autoimmune disorders
2. to diagnose Hashimoto's thyroiditis

**TSH (Thyrotropin)**
Thyrotropin is a hormone secreted by the anterior lobe of the pituitary that stimulates the thyroid gland. TSH test helps to distinguish between primary, secondary, and tertiary hypothyroidism by testing responsiveness of the anterior lobe of the pituitary gland.

*Indications:*
1. To diagnose hypothyroidism
2. To distinguish between primary and secondary hypothyroidism
3. To monitor patient response to thyroid replacement therapy

## Thyroid Scan
Thyroid scan is a radioisotope procedure, which provides information on the size, structure, position, and functioning of the thyroid gland.

*Indications:* To diagnose hyper—and hypothyroidism

## Thyroid ultrasonography
Thyroid ultrasonography aids in the non-invasive visualization of the thyroid gland in order to evaluate the structure and size of the thyroid gland. Ultrasonography is often done in conjunction with thyroid scans.

*Indications:*
1. to differentiate between a cyst and a tumor
2. to evaluate the size and structure of the thyroid gland

## Thyroxine (T4), serum
In increases the use of all food types for energy production and increases the rate of protein synthesis in most tissues.

*Indications:*
1. To evaluate thyroid function
2. To confirm the diagnosis of hyper—or hypothyroidism
3. To evaluate therapy for hyper—or hypothyroidism

## Serum T3
T3, in conjunction with T4, is useful in diagnosing hyperthyroidism. T3 is not usually utilized as a test for hypothyroidism.

*Indications:*
1. To determine hyper or hypothyroidism
2. To diagnose triidothyronine toxicosis

## Serum T4 or Thyroxine test
Most of the thyroid hormone secreted by the thyroid gland is in the form of T4, but T3 is the active hormone; i.e., T4 is converted to T3 by tissues in the body. T4 test or thyroxine test or thyroid function test is used to measure the amount of T4 in the blood.

*Indications:*
1. to evaluate thyroid function
2. to diagnose hyperthyroidism or hypothyroidism
3. to monitor thyroid replacement therapy

# GASTROINTESTINAL SYSTEM

### Abdominal X-ray
Abdominal X-ray aids in the diagnosis of gastrointestinal, hepatobiliary, and urological diseases.

*Indications:*
1. To identify changes in the position, size, contour, structure, and density of organs and tissues
2. To use for diagnosis, screening, or evaluation of healing
3. To identify abnormal air, fluid, and objects in the abdomen
4. To detect calcium deposits in cysts, tumors, blood vessels, and lymph nodes.
5. To evaluate kidneys, ureter and bladder
6. To diagnose urinary stones in kidney, ureter, bladder, or urethra
7. To detect gall stones
8. To detect bowel obstruction due to tumors, adhesions, hernia, or inflammation to detect foreign bodies

### Abdominal ultrasound
Abdominal ultrasound aids in the visualization of the specific abdominal organs or regions. It is frequently used to detect and monitor abdominal aneurysms.

*Indications*: to detect tumors, cysts, hypertrophy, abscesses, atherosclerotic plaques, obstruction or stricture, calculus, congenital anomaly, aneurysm, hematoma, foreign body, pregnancy, fetal development

### Barium enema
A barium enema is a radiological examination of the colon using barium instilled via a rectal tube into the rectum.

*Indications:*
1. to identify and locate benign or malignant polyps and tumors
2. to evaluate intussusception in children
3. to determine the cause of rectal bleeding, pus, or mucus in the feces

### Barium swallow
Barium swallow is radiographic examination of the esophagus during and after introduction of a contrast medium consisting of barium sulfate, which allows indirect visualization of the upper gastrointestinal system.

*Indications:*
1. to diagnose suspected strictures, diverticula, tumor, or polyps
2. to diagnose esophageal cancer, hiatal hernia diverticula, ulcers, and achalasia
3. to diagnose small bowel disorders, such as tumor, malabsorption syndrome, and inflammation

## Colonoscopy

Colonoscopy is the visualization of the lower gastrointestinal tract with insertion of a flexible endoscope through the anus to inspect the entire colon and terminal ileum. It is the most direct way to visualize the intestinal mucosa.

*Indications*
1. To diagnose polyps and tumors, colitis and diverticula
2. To identify and biopsy abnormal tissue in the colon and terminal ileum
3. To investigate the cause of chronic diarrhea
4. To locate the source of GI bleeding

## Computed Tomography, Abdomen

Computed axial tomography offers axial visualization of abdominal tissues. It images the cross sections of tissue structures.

*Indications:*
1. To diagnose abdominal aneurysms, hernias, ascites, abscesses, neoplasms
2. To diagnose trauma to the internal organs
3. To detect any abnormalities in the internal organs like adrenals, kidney, spleen, uterus, and biliary tract

## Computed Tomography, Pancreas

CT, Pancreas images cross sections of the tissue structures of the pancreas in conditions like acute pancreatitis.

*Indications:*
1. to diagnose acute pancreatitis
2. to detect any tumors or inflammatory growths

## Pancreas Scan:

It is a radioisotope scan that provides information on the structure and functioning of the pancreas.

*Indications:*
1. to detect pancreatic cancer
2. to detect pancreatic cysts

**Esophageal Acidity Test**
An esophageal acidity test aids in the assessment of esophageal sphincter's capability.

*Indications:*
To detect gastroesophageal reflux disease

**Esophagogastroduodenoscopy**
Esophagogastroduodenoscopy aids to visualize abnormalities in the esophagus, stomach, and duodenum.

*Indications:*
1. to diagnose tumors in the esophagus, stomach, and duodenum
2. to detect esophagitis, gastritis, duodenitis, ulcers and diverticula.
3. To take biopsy of suspected areas

**Proctosigmoidoscopy**
It aids in the visualization of the rectum and the lower part of the large intestine. It is similar to colonoscopy but not as extensive.

*Indications:*
1. to detect hemorrhoids
2. to detect polyps and abscesses
3. to determine the cause of bleeding

**Gallbladder Scan or HIDA scan**
Gallbladder scan aids to obtain images of the hepatobiliary system as an aid to the diagnosis of obstruction within the cystic and common bile ducts.

*Indications:*
1. To diagnose acute cholecystitis
2. To diagnose cystic and common bile duct obstruction

**Gastroscopy**
Gastroscopy aids in the visualization of entire esophagus, stomach, and proximal duodenum.

*Indications:*
1. To detect gastric bleeding
2. To detect gastric polyps
3. To detect gastric cancer

### Intrinsic Factor Antibody
This test measures the intrinsic factor, which is produced by the gastric cells of the stomach mucosa.

*Indications:*
To assess for anemia caused by a low B12 level

### Lactose Tolerance
A lactose tolerance test indicates the deficiency of intestinal disaccharide in the blood.

*Indications:*
1. To detect lactose intolerance
2. To identify irritable bowel syndrome

### Laparoscopy
Laparoscopy aids in the direct visualization of the anterior intra-abdominal structures with a laparoscope.

*Indications:*
1. to evaluate chronic abdominal pain
2. to detect ascites, suspected peritoneal carcinoma
3. to detect suspected ectopic pregnancy, salpingitis, hydrosalpinx, uterine fibroids, and infertility
4. evaluate adhesions, foreign bodies
5. to detect and monitor abscess formations

### Fecal Occult Blood Test—FOBT
Occult blood tests for the presence of blood in the stool to detect any gastrointestinal bleeding.

*Indications:*
1. to screen for carcinomas and polyps of GI tract
2. to detect GI bleeding

### Paracentesis
Peritoneal fluid analysis or paracentesis is used to remove accumulated exudative or transudative fluid from the abdominal cavity for diagnostic or therapeutic purposes.

*Indications:*
1. to diagnose infectious peritonitis
2. to detect the cause of ascites of uncertain origin
3. to identify bleeding into the peritoneal cavity

**Esophageal pH monitoring** or **Esophageal Acidity Test**
24-hour Ph monitoring is the gold standard test for the diagnosis of GERD. Esophageal acidity test is used to measure the frequency and duration of gastric acid that enters the esophagus. It is also useful to assess the function of lower esophageal sphincter.

*Indications:*
1. to assess the amount of gastric acid entering the esophagus and to evaluate it's clearance
2. to evaluate the absence or presence of GERD

**Rectal biopsy**
Rectal biopsy involves obtaining a small piece of rectal mucosa and submucosal tissue for microscopic examination.

*Indications:*
1. to diagnose rectal masses suspected of polyps or cancers
2. for the staging of Crohn's disease and ulcerative colitis
3. to diagnose Hirschsprung's disease and aganglionosis

**Secretin Stimulation Test for Zollinger-Ellison Syndrome**
Secretin stimulation test is used to measure the serum gastrin, which is produced in excessive amounts in Zollinger-Ellison syndrome.

*Indications:*
1. to diagnose Zollinger-Ellison syndrome
2. to evaluate ulcers, which are resistant to standard therapy.

**Sialography**
Sialography aids in the x-ray visualization of the salivary glands.

*Indications:*
1. to diagnose stones in the salivary ducts
2. to detect the cause of an enlarged salivary gland.

**Sigmoidoscopy**
A sigmoidoscopy aids in the direct visualization of the walls of the colon.

*Indications:*
1. to evaluate diverticular disease
2. to evaluate irritable bowel syndrome
3. to screen for colon cancer
4. to locate areas of bleeding and ulceration

**Stool culture**
Stool cultures are used to diagnose and monitor enteric pathogens.

*Indications:*
1. To detect parasites
2. To detect enteric disease causing pathogens and viruses

**Urea breath test**
Urea breath test is used to evaluate the presence of H.pylori

*Indications:*
To evaluate infection with H.pylori

**Vitamin B complex**
Vitamin B complex tests are used to test for vitamin levels that can detect many abnormalities or conditions.

*Indications:*
1. to detect Thiamine deficiency
2. to diagnose anemia due to vitamin deficiency

**Carcinoembryonic antigen**
Carcinoembryonic antigen is a molecular marker found on normal fetal cells and in the bloodstream of patients with cancers of the colon, breast, lung, and other organs.

*Indications:*
1. To monitor the effectiveness and success of cancer therapy
2. To provide prognostic information to the patient
3. To monitor for recurrence of cancer in the gastrointestinal tract, particularly colorectal cancer

# HEMATOLOGICAL SYSTEM

**APTT**
Activated Partial Throboplastin Time (APTT) is a sensitive-measure of blood-clotting ability. This test is very useful to monitor anticoagulation therapy.

*Indications:*
1. to diagnose inherited deficiency of blood-clotting factors
2. to diagnose liver disease
3. to diagnose Vitamin K deficiency
4. to diagnose Disseminated Intravascular Clotting deficiency

**Reticulocyte count**

Reticulocytes comprise 0.5 to 2.0% of total red-blood-cell count.

*Indications:*
1. Bone marrow disease
2. Hypoplastic anemia

**Alkaline Phosphatase**
Alkaline phosphatase is a group of enzymes found primarily in the liver, gallbladder, and intestinal and bone tissues. It is done primarily to assist in the diagnosis of hepatic and bone disease.

*Indications:*
1. to assist in the diagnosis of liver diseases
2. to assist in the diagnosis of bone diseases

**Alpha-Fetoprotein**
Alpha-fetoprotein is an antigen present in the human fetus and in certain pathological conditions in the adult.

*Indications:*
1. to detect anencephaly, encephalocele, spina bifida, myelomeningocele
2. to detect fetal renal abnormalities, multiple gestations
3. to detect esophageal and duodenal atresia

**Arterial Blood Gas Sampling**
Arterial blood gas testing measures the dissolved oxygen, carbon dioxide, and pH levels in the arterial blood.

*Indications:*
1. to detect ARDS, hypoxia, hypocapnia, congenital heart defects
2. to detect emphysema, pneumonia, sepsis, and shock

**Bleeding time**
Bleeding time is used as a screening procedure to evaluate the function of platelets and small blood vessels.

*Indications:*
1. to detect bleeding disorders
2. to evaluate DIC, liver disease, Hodgkin's disease etc.

**Blood culture**

Blood cultures are evaluated for the presence of bacteria in the blood.

*Indications:* to detect bacteremia

**Blood Group Antigen of Semen, Vaginal swab**

In rape victims, the blood type of the perpetrator may be identified by obtaining semen from the vagina of the rape victim.

*Indications*: rape trauma investigations

**Blood Typing and Cross-Matching**

Blood typing and cross-matching involve determining the four major blood types (A, B, AB, and O).

*Indications:*
1. to identify the patient's ABO type
2. to predict hemolytic disease in the newborn
3. to determine the need for immunosuppressive therapy after pregnancy

**Bone Marrow Examination**

Bone marrow examination involves removing bone marrow cells from the marrow and examining them to identify any pathological characteristics.

*Indications:*
1. to diagnose aplastic anemia, leukemia, lymphoma
2. to diagnose multiple myeloma, megaloblastic anemia, ITP, and iron deficiency anemia

**Carboxyhemoglobin**

Carboxyhemoglobin is a compound formed by carbon monoxide and hemoglobin in carbon monoxide poisoning.

*Indications:*
1. to evaluate smoke inhalation
2. to diagnose carbon monoxide poisoning

**Ceruloplasmin**

Ceruloplasmin is a blue glycoprotein to which most of the copper in the blood is attached. It is decreased in Wilson's disease

*Indications:*
1. to diagnose Wilson's disease
2. to detect copper intoxication

## Complete Blood Count

CBC is a combination report of a series of tests of the peripheral blood. The tests usually included in a CBC are hemoglobin, hematocrit, RBC count, RBC indices, WBC count, and differential WBC count.

*Indications:* in all cases which require information about hematological system

## Fibrin Degradation Products

This test is used to measure fibrin degradation products in blood.

*Indications:*
1. to evaluate the activity of the fibrinolytic system
2. to detect disseminated intravascular coagulation (DIC)

## Blood Alcohol level

Measuring blood alcohol level helps estimate alcohol intoxication.

*Indications:* To diagnose severity of alcohol ingestion

## Folic Acid

Folic acid is vitamin required for normal functioning of the red and white blood cells.

*Indications:* to detect Folic acid deficiency

## Glucose-6-Phosphate Dehydrogenase

G-6-PD deficiency is an inherited disorder that is transmitted as an autosomal recessive trait. G6PD screening is indicated for those most likely to have a defect.

*Indications:* to detect G-6-PD deficiency

## Ham's Test or Acid Hemolysis Test

It is a test for diagnosing paroxysmal nocturnal hemoglobinuria. In this test the red cells are assessed for resistance to lysis during incubation with acidified serum.

*Indication:*
1. to diagnose hemolytic anemia
2. to diagnose paroxysmal nocturnal hemoglobinuria

## Hematocrit

Hematocrit is the volume of erythrocytes packed by centrifugation in a given volume of blood. It is expressed as the percentage of total blood volume that consists of erythrocytes.

*Indications:*
1. as a part of CBC
2. to diagnose anemia

## Hemoglobin

Hemoglobin is the iron-containing pigment of red blood cells that carries oxygen from the lungs to the tissues.

*Indications:*
1. to diagnose anemia
2. to monitor blood loss

## Serum Iron

Serum Iron testing is used to assess for iron levels in the blood.

*Indications:*
1. to diagnose iron deficiency anemia
2. to detect iron toxicity

## Lactate Dehydrogenase

In humans, LD is present in several molecular forms called isoenzymes. A serum sample of LDH assists in diagnosing the amount of tissue damage.

*Indications:*
1. to diagnose suspected myocardial infarction
2. to diagnose anemia
3. to evaluate liver disorders

## Lead

Any level of lead in the blood is abnormal. Children who eat the paint develop signs of lead toxicity.

*Indications:*
1. to detect lead toxicity
2. to evaluate microcytic anemia

**Platelet Aggregation and Adhesion**
Platelet aggregation and adhesion tests measure the normal platelet function in coagulation.

*Indications*: to detect platelet disorders

**Platelet Count**
Platelet count measures the number of platelet cells.

*Indications:*
1. as a part of routine blood screen
2. to detect platelet diseases

**Serum Potassium**
A potassium test measures the amount of electrolyte potassium in the blood.

*Indications:*
To detect disorders that involve disturbances in potassium levels

**Serum Protein**
A serum protein test measures the total protein level in the blood.

*Indications:*
To diagnose diseases associated with altered serum protein levels.

**Prothrombin Time**
Prothrombin time evaluates the extrinsic pathway of coagulation.

*Indications:*
To detect the deficiency of coagulation factors

**Sickle Cell Test**
Sickle cell test is used to identify sickled cells in a blood sample.

*Indications:* to diagnose the presence of sickle cell anemia

**Von Willebrand Factor Assay**
Von Willebrand's disease is an inherited bleeding disorder, which affects coagulation factor 8.

*Indications:*
To detect von Willebrand's disease

# HEPATOBILIARY SYSTEM

### Alanine Aminotransferase—SGPT
Alanine aminotransferase is found in high concentration in liver cells, cardiac, renal, and skeletal tissues.

*Indications:* In the evaluation and monitoring of hepatic disorders

### Bilirubin
Bilirubin, a by-product of hemoglobin metabolism, is produced in the liver, spleen, and bone marrow.

*Indications:*
1.  in the evaluation of alcoholism
2.  to detect biliary diseases, hepatitis, cirrhosis, Gilbert's disease

### Intravenous Cholangiography
It is a contrast x-ray used to detect gallstones, obstructions, or other abnormalities of the gallbladder and bile ducts.

*Indications:* to identify stenosis, obstructions, and calculi of the common bile duct

### Cholecystography
It is a contrast x-ray study of the gallbladder.
*Indications:*
1.  To diagnose gallstones
2.  To diagnose gall bladder tumors and inflammatory diseases.

### Computed Tomography, Biliary Tract and Liver
Computed tomography can be used to provide images of the cross sections of liver and biliary tract.

*Indications:*
1.  to diagnose benign and malignant hepatic tumors and abscesses
2.  to detect biliary obstruction
3.  to detect cirrhosis, stenosis, and hepatitis

### Endoscopic Retrograde Cholangiopancreatography (ERCP)
ERCP is the x-ray visualization of the ducts leading from the pancreas and the gallbladder.

*Indications:* To diagnose the presence of stones or tumors in these ducts

**Hepatitis virus studies**
Viral hepatitis is any type of liver inflammation caused by a viral infection. There are five major types of viral hepatitis. These are hepatitis A, B, C, D, and E.

*Indication:*
To diagnose and monitor the course of viral hepatitis

**Liver Biopsy**
A liver biopsy is a procedure by which a thin core of liver tissue is obtained for analysis under a microscope.

*Indications:*
1. Chronic viral hepatitis like hepatitis B and hepatitis C
2. Alcohol induced liver disease
3. Drug induced liver damage
4. Space occupying liver lesions like tumors and cancers
5. Unexplained liver enlargement and liver tests
6. Storage diseases of liver
7. Systemic diseases and infections affecting the liver

**Liver Scan**
This is an isotope study, which provides information on the structure and functioning of the liver.

*Indications:*
1. Evaluation of size, shape, and position of liver
2. to detect cirrhosis
3. to detect liver abscesses, cysts and primary tumors
4. to diagnose liver tumors evaluation of patients with suspected liver rupture

**Percutaneous Transhepatic Cholangiography (PTCA)**
It is a contrast x-ray study of the bile duct, in which the contrast medium is administered through a needle directly into the liver.

*Indications:*
It is often used to diagnose causes of jaundice

**Spleen Scan**
Spleen scan uses a radioactive isotope to help determine spleen function.

*Indications:*
1. Evaluation of size, shape, and position of spleen

2. evaluation of patients with suspected spleen rupture
3. detection of space occupying lesions: abscesses, cysts, and primary tumors
4. detection of accessory splenic tissue or asplenia

**Urine Urobilinogen Test**
Urine urobilinogen is one of the most sensitive tests available to detect liver dysfunction.

*Indications:* to evaluate the liver function

# IMMUNOLOGICAL SYSTEM

**Allergen skin Testing**
Allergen skin testing is used to establish the allergies in the light of a positive clinical history. The choice of allergen (tree pollens, weeds, cat or dog dander, dust mites, metals like copper or nickel) extracts depends on the patient's allergy history.

*Indications:*
Patients presenting with symptoms suggestive of an allergic disorder, such as red, itching watery eyes, frequent post-nasal drip, sneezing, itchy, scratchy, or sore throat or asthma.

**Alpha-1 Antitrypsin**
Alpha-1 antitrypsin is an enzyme that is thought to inhibit the protease release from dead or dying cells. Its deficiency may result in such conditions like early-onset emphysema and liver dysfunction. The lower the level of normal AAT, the greater the risk of developing emphysema.

*Indications:*
1. to diagnose the cause of early onset emphysema
2. to diagnose the cause of persistent jaundice or other signs of liver dysfunction

**Anti-DNA Antibody**: Anti-DNA antibodies measure the presence of antibodies to native DNA. Anti-double-stranded DNA antibodies are commonly present in systemic lupus erythematosus.

*Indications*: to diagnose systemic lupus erythematosus

**Anti-La (SSB) & Anti-SS-A(Ro)**
Anti-La (SSB) and Anti-SS-A(Ro) are markers for Sjogren's syndrome.

*Indications:* to diagnose Sjogren's syndrome

**Antinuclear Antibody**
In certain autoimmune disorders antinuclear antibodies are produced and act against the body's own DNA and nuclear material resulting in pathological effects.

*Indications:*
To diagnose myasthenia gravis, Raynaud's syndrome, rheumatoid arthritis, SLE, and pulmonary fibrosis.

**AntiRNP**
Anti-RNP is an antinuclear antibody present in certain autoimmune disorders.

*Indications:* to diagnose scleroderma, discoid and systemic lupus erythematosus.

**Anti-Smooth Muscle Test**
Anti-smooth muscle test is an immunofluorescent test that can be ordered in conjunction with the test for antimitochondrial antibodies.

*Indications:* to differentiate between primary biliary cirrhosis and chronic active hepatitis

**Arylsulfatase A**
Arylsulfatase A is a lysosomal enzyme found in all body cells except mature RBCs.

*Indications:* to diagnose metachromatic leukodystrophy

**Bence Jones Protein**
Bence Jones Protein is a specific protein associated with multiple myeloma, macroglobulinemia, and malignant lymphoma.

*Indications:*
1. to detect multiple myeloma
2. to diagnose amyloidosis, Fanconi's syndrome, and Waldenstrom's macroglobulinemia

**Cold Agglutinins**
Cold agglutinins are usually IgM autoantibodies that are normally found in small amounts and indicate infection when increased.

*Indications:* to detect influenza, viral pneumonia, infectious mononucleosis etc.

**Enzyme-Linked Immunosorbent Assay**
ELISA detects antibodies that result from exposure to HIV.

*Indications:* to diagnose HIV infection

### Hepatitis B surface Antigen
Hepatitis B surface antigen is the earliest indicator of hepatitis B and its presence may indicate acute or chronic (carrier) hepatitis B.

*Indications:*
1. to screen for the presence of hepatitis B
2. to identify hepatitis B carrier state
3. to evaluate the progress of hepatitis management

### Western Blot Test or HIV Antibody
The Western blot assay is a test that determines the presence of antibodies for HTLV type 3 AIDS virus.

*Indications:* to confirm HIV infection with relative certainty

### Immunoglobulins
Immunoglobulin groups include IgA, IgD, IgE, IgG, IgM.

*Indications*: to detect serum immunoglobulin abnormalities

### Borrelia burgdorferi or Lyme disease test
The IgM antibodies produced in the body of Lyme disease patient can be detected by ELISA in the early stage and by the Western blot in the later stage.

*Indications:* to diagnose Lyme disease

### Lymphogranuloma Venereum Titer
LGV titer test allows for the detection of Chlamydia trachomatis serotypes L1, L2, and L3, which are the causative agents of Lymphogranuloma venereum.

*Indications*: to diagnose LGV

### Heterophile antibodies or Mononucleosis Spot Test
Detection of heterophile antibodies is the diagnostic test of choice in most clinical situations of suspected infectious mononucleosis

*Indications:* to detect infectious mononucleosis

**Rheumatoid Factor**
Rheumatoid Factor is an IgM antibody and is useful as a test for the detection of autoimmune disorders.

*Indications:* to diagnose rheumatoid arthritis

**Schick Test**
Schick test is a skin test that determines the degree of immunity to diphtheria.

*Indications:* to diagnose diphtheria

**Tests for Sexually Transmitted Disease**

**AIDS and HIV**
ELISA is the screening test for HIV infection while Western blot is the confirmatory test for HIV. CBC and CD4 lymphocyte counts are predictors of HIV progression. HIV viral load tests and p24 antigen tests can be indicated to measure the amount of actively replicating HIV virus. AIDS is a clinical, not a laboratory, diagnosis.

**Chlamydia**
Diagnosis is determined by blood tests, culturing, Direct immunofluorescence assay, enzyme-linked immunoassay, DNA probe tests, Ligase chain reaction etc.

**Genital herpes**
Diagnosis is made by culturing blood from lesions.

**Gonorrhea**
Culture is the gold standard for diagnosis of gonorrhea. Ligase Chain Reaction (LCR) detects both N gonorrhea and Chlamydia trachomatis, and permits more rapid diagnosis of gonococcal infection.

**Syphilis**
RPR and VDRL are used as screening tests for syphilis. Positive results indicate the need for a confirmatory test (FTA-ABS and MHA-TP)

**Throat cultures**
In throat cultures, material from the posterior pharynx is obtained through swabbing and examined to identify the bacteria.

*Indications:* to identify the bacteria or virus in the patients with pharyngitis

**Viral culture**
Though viruses are not routinely cultured because of the limited availability of anti-viral therapies it is useful for early detection of viral infection. A viral culture is used to identify a viral infection.

*Indications:* to diagnose viral diseases

**White Blood Cell Count and Differential Count**
WBC and differential count are performed to determine the amount of WBCs in the blood.

*Indications:*
1. to evaluate the changes in WBC count
2. to know the type of WBC involved in patient's hematological responses.

# INTEGUMENTARY SYSTEM

**Skin culture**
Skin cultures are useful to detect the presence of abnormal microorganisms in the sample of the infected area.

*Indications:* to identify the organisms responsible for a skin abscess, carbuncle, impetigo, erysipelas, warts, dermatophytes, tinea cruris and other skin lesions.

**Sweat Test**
Sweat test is a diagnostic test for cystic fibrosis, which measures the chloride present in sweat.

*Indications:* to diagnose cystic fibrosis

**Tzanck Test**
Tzanck test is a rapid method of determining the nature of cells in blistering diseases of the skin such as herpes virus lesions or pemphigus vulgaris

**Radio-Allergosorbent Test (RAST)**
RASTs are useful in the diagnosis of conditions like extrinsic asthma, hay fever, and atopic eczema

*Indications:* to identify the patient's reactivity to a specific allergen

# LYMPHATIC SYSTEM

### Lymphangiography
Lymphangiography is a contrast x-ray procedure, which aids in the diagnosis of the swelling in the legs and feet, and the presence of cancer in the lymphatic system.

*Indications:* to detect lymphedema and lymphoma metastatic disease

### Retroperitoneal Ultrasonography
Retroperitoneal ultrasonography is used to evaluate retroperitoneal organ sizes and pathological states, such as lymphoma and metastatic spread of cancer.

*Indications:* Retroperitoneal ultrasonography can be used to identify cysts and other collections of fluid, structural defects, tumors, and vascular lesions in the retroperitoneal areas.

### Spleen Sonogram
Spleen sonogram involves an ultrasound probe of the spleen.

*Indications:*
1.  to evaluate splenic abnormalities such as masses, cysts, and splenomegaly.
2.  to evaluate damage to spleen from abdominal trauma

# METABOLIC SYSTEM

### Ammonia
Ammonia is produced in the liver, intestine, and kidneys as the end product of protein metabolism.

*Indications:* to monitor liver function and metabolism

### Amylase
Amylase is an enzyme synthesized in the pancreas and salivary glands and secreted into the gastrointestinal tract, which helps digest starch and glycogen in the mouth, stomach, and intestine.

*Indications:* to diagnose acute pancreatitis

### Benedict's Test
Benedict's test is used to screen for presence of sugars, reducing substances, and homogentisic acids in the urine.

*Indications:* to diagnose ochronosis

### Pancreatic Sonogram
Ultrasonography of the pancreas to identify the abnormalities in the pancreas

*Indications:* To detect tumors, cysts or pseudocysts in the pancreas

### Hemosiderin
Hemosiderin measures the presence of iron storage granules in urine sediment. The finding of hemosiderin is indicative of extensive hemolysis, iron metabolism disorder or renal tubular damage.

*Indications:*
1. to detect the etiology of RBC hemolysis
2. to evaluate renal tubule dysfunction

# MUSCULOSKELETAL SYSTEM

### MRI Scan
MRI is a non-invasive procedure that uses powerful magnets and radio waves to construct pictures of the body.

*Indications:* MRI scans are excellent in spine, joint, and soft-tissue imaging. It offers the advantage of seeing soft-tissue detail and often identifies the extent of sarcomas.

**Acetylcholine Receptor-Binding Antibodies**: Acetyl choline receptor antibodies are a family of antibodies that develops in myasthenia gravis, a disease that affects the transmission of nerve impulses.

*Indication:* to diagnose myasthenia gravis

### Aldolase Test
Aldolast test is used to measure the amount of the enzyme aldolase in serum. Aldolase is an enzyme present in skeletal and heart muscle and the liver. It is involved in the breakdown of glucose, fructose, and galactose. Aldolase is in a particularly high concentration in muscle

*Indication:* to evaluate the muscle damage

### Arthrography
Arthrography is a technique of injecting contrast material into the joint to evaluate joint capsule and articular surface integrity. It aids in the x-ray visualization of the joint.

*Indications:* Rotator cuff tears in the shoulder, interrosseous ligament tears at the wrist, knee meniscal tears.

**Arthroscopy**
Direct joint visualization by means of a fiber-optic endoscope, usually to remove tissue, such as cartilage fragments or torn ligaments, or to anneal injured tissues.

*Indications:*
1. to diagnose various joint diseases
2. to perform surgery on the joint

**Bone Marrow Scan**
*Indications:*
1. to evaluate regional bone marrow abnormalities
2. to assess suspected areas of avascular necrosis
3. to diagnose osteomyelitis
4. to identify marrow replacement by tumor

**Bone Scan**
A bone scan is a radioisotope technique indicative of blood flow and thereby of bone formation or destruction.

*Indications:* to identify infection, bone tumors, degenerative bone diseases, trauma and fractures.

**Computed Tomography Scan**
CT Scan offers axial visualization of bone, muscle, and fat tissues. Bone visualization is usually excellent than soft-tissue structures.

*Indication:* to visualize complex fracture patterns, especially with joint involvement.

**C Reactive Protein**
C-reactive protein (CRP) is the only inflammatory marker that has been found to be an indicator of cardiac health. The C-reactive protein (CRP) test is a blood test that measures the level of CRP in the blood.

*Indications:*
1. to predict a patient's risk of a heart attack
2. to predict coronary artery disease and stroke
3. to evaluate the course of atherosclerosis and stenosis
4. To help with the diagnosis of Rheumatoid Arthritis and Rheumatic Fever

**Electromyography**
Electromyography is the graphic record of resting and voluntary muscle activity as a result of electrical stimulation.

*Indications:*
1. to diagnose muscular diseases
2. to detect peripheral nerve disorders
3. to detect spinal cord disorders

## Electroneurography
Electroneurography is the measurement of the conduction velocity and latency of peripheral nerves.

*Indications:*
1. To investigate neuromuscular disorders such as peripheral neuropathy caused by diabetes or alcoholism
2. to investigate primary muscle diseases like muscular dystrophy, myasthenia gravis
3. to investigate secondary muscle diseases like polymyositis, sarcoidosis, tetanus etc.
4. to evaluate myopathies or neuropathies

## Myelogram
Myelogram is a radiograph of the spinal cord and associated nerves. This procedure aids in the visualization of the spinal subarachnoid space—the area between the spinal cord and the arachnoid membrane that covers it.

*Indications:*
1. to diagnose herniated disks
2. to diagnose spinal nerve injury
3. to detect spinal tumors

## Urine Myoglobin Test
Myoglobin is a protein in heart and skeletal muscles. It is the iron-containing protein found in muscle cells that stores oxygen for use in cell respiration. This is a test to detect the presence of myoglobin in urine. Increased levels of myoglobin are found with myocardial infarction, muscular dystrophy, polymyositis, and renal failure.

*Indications:*
Myoglobin tests are done to evaluate a person who has symptoms of myocardial infarction or other muscle damage.

## Radiography
They are the mainstay of bone and joint imaging.

*Indications:*
Deformity of a bone or joint

Inability to use a limb or joint

Unexplained pain in a bone or joint

## Sinus Endoscopy

Sinus endoscopy aids in the visualization of the mucosal surface of the sinuses using an endoscope.

*Indications:* to identify inflammation, tumors or other anatomic changes in the sinuses

## Sinus X-ray

Sinus X-ray involves x-ray of the sinuses that aid in the diagnosis of sinusitis.

*Indications:*

1. to diagnosis acute or chronic sinusitis
2. to evaluate obstruction of nasal sinuses
3. to detect sinus tumors or abscesses

## Skull X-ray

X-ray of the skull.

*Indications:*

1. to diagnose skull fractures
2. to evaluate head injury
3. to discover radiopaque tumors

## Spinal X-ray

Spinal X-ray involves the radiography of cervical, thoracic, and lumbosacral spine areas to detect spinal abnormalities such as fractures and masses.

*Indications:*

1. to assess back or neck pain
2. to evaluate scoliosis or lordosis
3. to evaluate congenital spinal cord defects
4. to diagnose spinal fractures
5. to diagnose spinal tumors

## Synovial Fluid Analysis

Synovial fluid analysis is a microscopic test of synovial fluid for clarity, percent of neutrophils, and WBC count.

*Indications:*
1.  to diagnose rheumatic disease
2.  to identify joint infections
3.  to evaluate joint inflammations

**Bone biopsy (bone needle aspiration cytology)**

*Indications:* To detect malignant bone tumors (osteogenic sarcoma, Ewing's sarcoma etc) and benign bone tumors (Giant cell tumors, Osteoma)

# NEUROLOGICAL SYSTEM

**Brain Scan**
Brain scan is a radioisotope study of the brain.

*Indications:*
1.  to detect brain tumors
2.  to diagnose brain hemorrhages, stroke
3.  to detect cerebral blood vessel abnormalities

**Brain Ultrasound**
Brain ultrasound is a noninvasive test that uses ultrasound waves to identify occlusions of the cerebral veins and arteries.

*Indications:* to evaluate and monitor hydrocephalus, abnormal bleeding in the brain, and cystic or solid tumors

**Cerebral Angiography**
Radiography of cerebral blood vessels, which is virtually similar to the angiography of the heart.

*Indications:*
1.  to locate the aneurysms
2.  to detect blood clots
3.  to detect other abnormalities, which cause stroke

**CSF Examination**
CSF is a watery cushion that protects the brain and spinal cord from physical impact and bathes the brain in electrolyte and proteins. Lumbar puncture provides a small amount of cerebrospinal fluid for laboratory analysis.

*Indications:*
1. to diagnose viral or bacterial infections
2. to detect brain hemorrhage

## CT Brain
CT Scanning is more sensitive than an MRI would be for the diagnosis of Subarachnoid hemorrhage.

## CT Spine
CT Spine involves cross-sectional imaging technology allows the radiologist to look at different levels or slices of the lower back using a rotating X-ray beam.

*Indications:* evaluate the cervical, thoracic, and lumbar spine.

## EEG
A tracing of the electrical activity of the brain.

*Indications:*
1. to diagnose epilepsy
2. to diagnose brain tumors

## Nerve Biopsy
A biopsy used to evaluate nerve disorders.

*Indications:* to evaluate primary or secondary neuropathies or systemic diseases like Amyloidosis

## Nerve Conduction Studies
Nerve conduction studies are useful in assessing a nerve's ability to carry a neural impulse and its speed of transmission.

*Indications:*
1. carpal tunnel syndrome
2. diabetic neuropathy
3. neuromuscular conditions
4. Muscle weakness, myopathy and myositis
5. Neuritis and nerve root compression
6. Spinal cord injury
7. Peripheral nerve disorders

## Tensilon Test
Tensilon test is used to detect any abnormalities in the neuromuscular junction.

*Indications:*
To diagnose myasthenia gravis

**Visual Evoked Response**
VER is a reaction produced in response to visual stimuli. While the patient is watching a pattern projected on a screen, the electroencephalogram is produced.

*Indications:*
1. to confirm the dianosis of multiple sclerosis
2. to diagnose optic nerve disorders
3. to detect brain and spinal cord tumors and abnormalities

# PULMONARY SYSTEM

**Sputum Acid-Fast Bacterial Culture and Stain**: Positive staining for acid-fast bacteria indicates the presence of Mycobacterium species.

*Indication:* to diagnose Tuberculosis

**Bronchoscopy**
Examination of the bronchi through a bronchoscope.

*Indications:*
1. to check for tumors or foreign bodies
2. to locate the site of internal bleeding
3. to remove mucus or a foreign body
4. to obtain a tissue or secretion specimen

**Bronchography**
Bronchography is an x-ray of the trachea and the bronchial tree.

*Indications:*
1. to help locate obstructions
2. to detect tumors and cysts in the bronchial tube

**Chest Radiography**
Chest radiography is one of the most commonly used tests to detect the abnormalities of lungs, pleura, thorax, soft tissues, heart and mediastinum.

*Indications:*
1. to detect pneumonia, lung abscess, pneumothorax, pericardial and pleural effusions

2.   to evaluate trauma to bony thorax
3.   to detect cardiac enlargement

## CT Chest

CT chest is useful to get the images of the cross sections of chest structures.

*Indications:*
1.   to evaluate lymphoma, bronchogenic carcinoma, sarcoma
2.   to detect metastatic lung cancers
3.   to evaluate chest trauma
4.   to diagnose pleural effusion

## Sputum Cytology

Sputum cytology is useful to determine the type and number of cells present in the sputum in order to diagnose pulmonary disorders.

*Indications:*
1.   to detect benign and malignant tumors
2.   to diagnose viral and fungal infections of the lungs
3.   to detect asbestosis, emphysema and other inflammatory lung disorders
4.   to evaluate metaplastic changes in the pulmonary tissues

## Laryngoscopy

Laryngoscopy involves the visual examination of the interior the larynx to determine the cause of hoarseness, obtain cultures, manage the upper airway, or take biopsies.

*Indications:*
1.   to detect foreign bodies in larynx
2.   to detect tumors in the larynx

## Lung Biopsy

Lung biopsy is used to obtain lung tissue, which can be used to examine for the presence of both benign and malignant lung diseases.

*Indications:* to diagnose interstitial fibrosis, sarcoidosis, and benign and malignant lung tumors

## Lung Scan

There are two types of lung scans: ventilation and perfusion.

*Indications:*
1.   to detect pulmonary embolism

2. to detect lung tumors
3. to evaluate emphysema

## Oximetry
Oximetry involves the use of an oximeter to determine the oxygen saturation of blood.

*Indications:*
1. to evaluate patients with respiratory compromise
2. to monitor for oxygen levels on perioperative and postoperative patients.

## Paranasal Sinus Films
Paranasal sinus films are indicated to determine the presence of abnormalities in sinus shape and structure.

*Indications:*
1. To diagnose acute or chronic sinusitis
2. To detect benign or malignant tumors or cysts in the sinuses
3. To detect abnormalities in the shape and structure of sinus

## Pleural Biopsy
Pleural biopsy involves obtaining a small pleural tissue sample through a transthoracic needle biopsy procedure (TTNB) and analyzing the tissue to detect pleural disorders.

*Indications:*
1. to diagnose pleural tumors
2. to diagnose pleural infections
3. to diagnose pleural fibrosis and collagen vascular disorders

## Pulmonary Function Tests
Pulmonary function tests are used to obtain data on the lung volumes, pattern, and air flow rates involved in respiratory function.

*Indications:*
1. to determine the cause of shortness of breath
2. to detect pulmonary diseases
3. to evaluate the patient before surgery
4. to evaluate disability for insurance purposes

## Spirometry
Spirometry is the most commonly indicated pulmonary function test, which involves measurement of air flow and lung volumes.

*Indications:*
1.  to diagnose asthma, emphysema, myasthenia gravis, bronchitis, and COPD
2.  to assess damage from smoking
3.  to evaluate the severity of asthma

**Mediastinoscopy**
Mediastinoscopy aids in the direct visualization of the tissues and organs in the thorax behind sternum.

*Indications:*
1.  to detect and evaluate various types of mediastinal cancers
2.  to evaluate infections in the thorax

# RENAL/UROLOGICAL SYSTEM

**Albumin**
Albumin is the smallest protein in blood, the presence of which in the urine is an indicator of renal disease.

*Indications:*
1.  to evaluate renal disorders like glomerulonephritis, nephritis, pyelonephritis
2.  to detect nephropathy in the patients with diabetes

**Bladder Ultrasonography**
Bladder ultrasonography involves the use of ultrasound to produce an image or photograph of bladder to examine the bladder's position, shape, and size.

*Indications:*
To diagnose bladder or pelvis tumors
To diagnose cancer of the bladder
To evaluate urinary tract obstruction

**Blood Urea Nitrogen**
Nitrogen in the blood in the form of urea, the metabolic product of the breakdown of amino acids used for energy production. The normal concentration is about 8 to 18 mg/dl.

*Indications:*
To evaluate renal function
To monitor patients in renal failure or those receiving dialysis therapy

## Catecholamines
Catecholamines include the biologically active amines derived from the amino acid tyrosine: metanephrine, dopamine, epinephrine and norepinephrine.

*Indications:*
To detect pheochromocytoma

## Renal CT Scan
CT Scan of the kidneys.

*Indications:* to provide information on the size, shape, and position of the kidneys.

## Serum Creatinine
Creatinine is the decomposition product of the metabolism of phosphocreatine, a source of energy for muscle contraction. The average normal serum creatinine value is less than 1.2 mg/dL.

*Indications:*
To evaluate disorders of kidney function, urinary obstruction, acromegaly, diabetes mellitus and thyroid disorders

## Cystography
Cystography involves the radiography of the bladder in which a contrast medium has been instilled.

*Indications:*
To diagnose neurogenic bladder, vesicoureteral reflux, bladder diverticula, fistulas between the bladder and adjacent organs

## Cystometry
Cystometry can be used to assess the neuromuscular function of the bladder when there are incontinence problems.

*Indications:*
1.  to evaluate bladder hypertonicity, urinary obstructions, and neurogenic bladder
2.  to determine bladder capacity
3.  to diagnose prostatic obstruction and urinary incontinence

**Glomerular Basement Membrane Antibody**
Anti-Glomerular basement membrane antibodies are present in the patient with Goodpasture's syndrome.

*Indications:* to diagnose Goodpasture's syndrome

**Introvenous Pyelography**
It involves radiography of the renal pelvis and ureter after injection of a radiopaque contrast medium. It provides visualization of the kidneys, ureters, and bladder.

*Indications:*
1. to evaluate the functioning of the kidneys and urinary tract
2. to detect renal calculi, tumors, polycystic kidney disease, hydronephrosis, ureteral calculi, urinary retention, and trauma

**Kidney Biopsy**
Kidney biopsy is used to obtain a tissue from the kidney for examination.

*Indications:*
To diagnose glomerulonephritis, pyelonephritis, kidney transplant rejections, renal cell carcinoma, Wilm's tumor and disseminated lupus erythematosus

**Oxalate**
Oxalate is a salt of oxalic acid. The amount of oxalate in the urine determines the formation of calcium oxalate calculi—kidney stones.

*Indications:* to diagnose primary hyperoxaluria, acquired hyperoxaluria and idiopathic hyperoxaluria

**Protein Electrophoresis**
Protein electrophoresis is used to measure the quantitative amount of proteins in the urine.

*Indications:*
1. to detect Bence Jones proteinuria, which is a symptom of multiple myeloma and monoclonal gammopathies
2. to diagnose glomerular and tubular renal disease

**Renal Angiography**
Renal angiography involves the radiography of the blood vessels and tissues of the kidney.

*Indications:*
1. to diagnose renal artery stenosis
2. to evaluate renal artery aneurysms, emboli, and hematoma

## Urine Toxicology Screening

Urine toxicology screening evaluates urine for the presence of legal and illegal drugs.

*Indications:*
1. to evaluate suspected drug use
2. to diagnose drug toxicity in unconscious or comatose patients

## Urethrography

Urethrography is radiography of the urethra after it has been filled with contrast medium. It provides a direct view of the urethra.

*Indications:* to diagnose urinary tract disorders

## Retrograde Urethrography

Retrograde urethrography is the contrast x-ray visualization of the front part of the urethra. It is done almost exclusively in males. A catheter is inserted into the urethra, through which the contrast medium is injected and X-rays are taken of the patient.

*Indications:* to diagnose injuries or abnormalities in the urethra.

## Voiding Cystourethrography

Voiding cystourethrography provides an x-ray picture of the bladder and urethra during urination.

*Indications:* to diagnose urinary tract disorders

## Blood Uric Acid

Uric acid is the end product of purine metabolism. It must be excreted because it cannot be metabolized.

*Indications:*
To diagnose gout, renal disease, starvation, alcoholism, psoriasis etc

## Urinalysis

Urinalysis is the analysis of the urine for the presence of blood, pus, glucose, hemoglobin, nitrites, bacteria, ketones, WBCs, casts and crystals. It involves examination of the urine by physical or chemical means.

*Indications:*
1. To diagnose diabetes, calculi, infections, and hemorrhages
2. To screen for urinary tract infections, renal disease, and diseases of other organs that result in abnormal metabolites appearing in the urine.

**Water Deprivation**

Water deprivation test to demonstrate that the patient's kidneys are capable of regulating urine output in response to low water intake. It tests the body's ability to concentrate urine when plasma osmolality is artificially increased.

*Indications:* to diagnose diabetes insipidus to detect abnormalities of osmolality of the body

**Water Loading**

Water loading test aids in the determination of water and electrolyte disturbances.

*Indications:*
1. to diagnose ADH secreting tumors
2. to evaluate dehydration, edema, ascites, cirrhosis, and CHF

# REPRODUCTIVE SYSTEM

**Amniocentesis:** A procedure in which fluid is obtained from the amniotic cavity by an ultrasound-guided needle (usually at weeks 15-17 of pregnancy) and analyzed for the presence of fetal abnormalities. It can be used to test for birth defects and to rule out Down syndrome, Tay-Sachs disease, neural tube disorders like spina bifida, and amino acid disorders.

*Indications:*
1. 3+ spontaneous abortions
2. maternal age greater than 35
3. previous history of chromosomally abnormal child
4. metabolic disease
5. neural tube defect
6. patient, father, or family history of chromosome abnormality
7. possible carrier of X-linked disease

**Breast Biopsy**
Breast biopsy is the obtaining of a representative tissue sample of breast for microscopic examination, usually to establish a diagnosis.

*Indications:*
1. to diagnose breast cancer
2. to evaluate abscesses, fibrocystic disease, cysts, and mastitis

## Cervical Culture
A cervical culture is performed to identify the etiological agents of cervicitis.

*Indications:*
1. to diagnose genital ulcers
2. to diagnose the cause of STDs
3. to evaluate abnormal discharges

## Chlamydia Test
A chlamydia infection is caused by chlamydia trachomatis bacteria and is the most common sexually transmitted disease in the United States.

*Indications:*
1. Patients presenting with a pus-like discharge from the penis or vagina, burning during urination, or pelvic pain
2. Men involved in unprotected sex and presenting with symptoms suggestive of chlamydial infection
3. Women involved in unprotected sex and presenting with symptoms suggestive of cervicitis, salpingitis, and pelvic inflammatory disease

## Chorionic Villus Sampling
It is a procedure for obtaining a sample of the chorionic villi, the examination of which is useful in prenatal evaluation of the chromosomal, enzymatic, and DNA status of the fetus. It can be done in early in pregnancy to test for damaged chromosomes.

*Indications:*
To detect serious fetal chromosomal abnormalities

## Colposcopy
Colposcopy aids in the direct visualization of the vagina and cervix.

*Indications:*
1. To evaluate an abnormal Pap smear (Papanicolaou's test)
2. To monitor for precancerous abnormalities
3. To evaluate a lesion of the vagina or cervix
4. To perform a biopsy

## Culdoscopy

Culdoscopy involves examination of the viscera of the female pelvic cavity after introduction of an endoscope through the wall of the posterior fornix of the vagina.

*Indications:*
1. to detect ectopic pregnancy, fallopian abnormalities, or pelvic masses
2. to identify ovarian cysts, uterine fibroids, or malignancies
3. to detect endometriosis, pelvic inflammatory disease

## Fetal Nonstress Test

Fetal nonstress testing (NST) is a noninvasive test that measures the fetal heart rate as it responds to fetal movement.

*Indications:*
1. to detect fetal stress
2. to confirm fetal death

## Fetoscopy

Fetoscopy involves direct visualization of the fetus in the uterus through a fetoscope.

*Indications:*
1. to detect fetal developmental defects
2. to diagnose blood dyscrasias of fetus

## Human Chorionic Gonadotropin

HCG is a hormone secreted by the placenta and can be detected in urine or serum within 10 days after the conception.

*Indications:*
1. to confirm pregnancy
2. to diagnose HCG-producing tumors, such as choriocarcinoma or hydatiform moles
3. to confirm threatened or incomplete abortion

## Hysterosalpingography

Hysterosalpingography of the uterus and fallopian tubes is use to detect abnormalities or obstructions in the fallopian tubes that may be the cause of infertility. This aids to explore the internal configuration of the uterine cavity.

*Indications:*
1. to identify uterine abnormalities
2. to assess the patency of the fallopian tubes

**Hysteroscopy**
It involves inspection of the uterus by use of a special endoscope.

*Indications:*
1. to diagnose uterine fibroids or adhesions
2. to evaluate endocervical tissues

**Infertility screen**
Infertility is the inability to achieve pregnancy during a year or more of unprotected intercourse. Infertility screen involves semen analysis for men to assess sperm morphology, motility and number. Female assessment is done initially with evaluation of ovulation by use of a basal body temperature graph. Additional special tests include evaluations of ovarian, tubal, uterine, and cervical factors.

*Indications:* for all couples who fail to achieve pregnancy during a year or more of unprotected intercourse.

**Mammography:** The radiologic examination of the breast using a special imaging device. It differs from a general X-ray exam in that it uses low energy X-rays to get high resolution and high contrast images of soft tissue. Mammography is the most effective way to detect breast cancer early. Mammography can find 85-90% of all breast cancer, making it the most reliable screening test.

Mammography is the single best noninvasive procedure for detecting breast cancer.
*Indications:*
1. to detect breast cancer
2. Skin change over the breast
3. Thickening of the breast
4. Breast lump
5. Suspicious nipple discharge

**Papanicolaou Smear:** Pap smear is a normal component of a gynecological examination and the best method to detect early, curable stages of malignancy as well as fungal, viral, and other infections of the female genital tract.

*Indications*: Pap smear is indicated as a standard screening method for early detection of HPV (Human Papilloma Virus), herpes, or trichomonad infections, cervical intraepithelial neoplasia(CIN or dysplasia), and carcinoma of cervix.

**Kleihauer-Betke Test**: This test is most commonly used to differentiate between fetal and maternal red blood cells in the mother's circulation or in amniotic fluid. It is used to estimate the volume of transplacental hemorrhage in mothers with Rh immune disease and the amount of Rh immune globulin that should be administered to the mother to reduce sensitization to Rh factor and to the child to reduce the incidence of Rh factor-induced hemolytic disease of the newborn.

*Indications in Step-2 CS:*
To determine the amount of Rh immune globulin an Rh-negative woman must receive to prevent her from developing antibodies against her fetus.

## Pelvic Sonogram
Pelvic sonogram involves visualization of the pelvis through the use of ultrasonography.

*Indications:*
1. to determine the stage of fetal development
2. to confirm the presence of more than one fetus
3. to determine the position of the fetus or placenta
4. to diagnose vaginal bleeding or any abnormal discharge
5. to guide the needle for amniocentesis
6. to detect pelvic masses
7. to detect uterine fibromas, cysts
8. to detect ovarian cysts

## Pelvimetry
Pelvimetry involves the measurement of pelvic dimensions or proportions, which helps determine whether or not it will be possible to deliver a fetus through the normal route.

## Postcoital test
It is done subsequent to sexual intercourse. It can be used as part of an infertility work-up. In this test, endocervical mucus is examined after coitus to detect its quality and the ability of the sperm to penetrate the mucus.

*Indications:*
1. to evaluate infertility
2. to evaluate rape cases for the presence of sputum

## Prolactin
Prolactin is a hormone produced by the anterior pituitary gland. It is elevated in many conditions such as addition's disease, anorexia nervosa, galactorrhea, acromegaly etc.

*Indications:*
1. to diagnose pituitary tumor
2. to evaluate oligorrhea, amenorrhea, or galactorrhea in women

3. to diagnose prolactin-secreting ectopic tumor of the lungs or kidneys
4. to evaluate impotence in men
5. to diagnose pituitary infarction

## Prostate Biopsy
Prostate biopsy is an invasive procedure in which a small tissue sample is taken from the prostate for microscopic examination.

*Indications:*
1. to diagnose prostate cancer
2. to diagnose prostate hypertrophy of unknown cause

## Prostate Sonogram
Prostate sonogram can be used to evaluate the size and consistency of the prostate tissue.

*Indications:*
1. to diagnose prostate cancer, prostate abscess, and perirectal abscess
2. for the staging of prostate cancer

## Prostate-Specific Antigen
Prostate-specific antigen tests for the levels of a serum protease enzyme specific to the male prostate.

*Indications:*
1. to diagnose prostate cancer in conjunction with the digital rectal examination

## Rapid Plasma Reagin
Reagin is the antibody specific to the Treponema pallidum spirochete. A rapid plasma reagin is the test that measures the amount of reagin in the plasma.

*Indications:*
To diagnose syphilis in secondary stage

## Rosette Test
Rosette test or fetal-maternal blood test is performed to detect fetal cells in the maternal circulation.

*Indications:* to detect fetal red blood cells in the maternal blood to detect anemia in the fetus

## Semen Analysis
Semen analysis can be ordered as part of an infertility work-up.

*Indications:*
1. to determine male infertility
2. to investigate suspected rape cases

**Testosterone**
Testosterone is a steroid sex hormone that is responsible for the growth and development of masculine characteristics.

*Indications*
1. in women complaining of hirsutism
2. in women suspected of having adrenal neoplasms, ovarin tumors, hilar cell tumor
3. in men suspected of having adrenal tumors, hyperthyroidism, idiopathic CNS tumor

**Vaginal Culture**
A vaginal culture is used to identify organisms present in the vagina.

*Indications:* to diagnose vaginal infections like trichomonas, herpes simplex, chlamydia, gonorrhea etc.

**VDRL Test**: Venereal Disease Research Laboratory Test

*Indications*: as screening test for syphilis.

**Note:** a positive VDRL test must be confirmed with FTA-ABS.

# SENSORY SYSTEM

**Electronystagmography**
Electronystagmography is a method of recording the electrical activity of the extraocular muscles.

*Indications:*
1. to assess dizziness, vertigo, brainstem lesions, cerebellum lesions
2. to diagnose different types of nystagmus
3. to diagnose the etiology of hearing loss

**Electroretinography**
Electroretinography involves a record of the action currents of the retina produced by visual or light stimuli.

*Indications:*
1. to diagnose retinal detachment, retinal damage, and retinitis
2. to detect congenital abnormalities that affect the corneal lens and retina

## Ocular Cytology

Ocular cytology is the microscopic examination of cell specimen taken from the eye.

*Indications:*
1. to diagnose intraocular and orbital tumors
2. to diagnose malignant conjunctival lesions

## Otoscopy

Otoscopy involves examination of the ear using an otoscope. It aids in the visualization of the external canal of the ear and the middle ear.

*Indications:* to identify the lesions of the external ear canal

## Slit-Lamp Biomicroscopy

It is a noninvasive visualization of the anterior portion of the eye and its parts.

*Indications:* to diagnose corneal abrasions, corneal ulcers, and cataracts

**Tonometry**: It is a technique that measures intraocular pressure (in mm Hg) by contact or noncontact on the eyeball.

*Indications*: to diagnose glaucoma and ocular hypertension and in routine ocular examination.

## Visual Acuity

Visual acuity is measure of the resolving power of the eye. It is usually determined by one's ability to read letters of various sizes at a standard distance from the test chart. Visual acuity is expressed as a fraction.

*Indications:* to assess overall visual acuity in all patients presenting with eye problems

# 9

## ✈ FREQUENTLY ASKED QUESTIONS ✈

## TEST SCHEDULING

*Is it possible to reschedule my testing appointment?*
Yes, you can reschedule your testing appointments as many times as you want, but it depends on the size of your wallet and the space on your calendar. You have to pay a rescheding fee.

*Can I exchange my test date with another student preparing for CS examination?*
Theoretically possible. But some students are making it a business. I do not advise it. Be careful

*Is Step-2 CK needed to take Step-2 CS?*
Step-2 CK is not needed to register for Step-2 CS. However, it helps you to form differential diagnosis and diagnostic work up easily. If you are comfortable in those areas you do not need to wait until you take Step-2 CK to go for Step-2 CS.

*I am an international medical student from Pakistan. English is not my mother language. Do I need to pass TOEFL to register for a clinical skills examination?*
Unlike for CSA, which required TOEFL passing score, for Step-2 CS you do not need to pass TOEFL. Your English will be tested under Spoken English Proficiency, one of the components of Step-2 CS Test.

*How long does it take to get an appointment for Step-2 CS?*
Once you send your application to NBME or ECFMG, they will respond within 3 weeks. Test spot availability varies from 4-6 months depending on the time of the year. But, getting a date during the months of July to January may be difficult because of the concomitance of ERAS during these months.

*I am an international medical graduate. How long would it take for the ECFMG to accept the Step-2 CS result for my ECFMG certificate?*
2-3 weeks

*When should I take the exam, morning or afternoon?*
It does'nt matter if you prepare well.

# TEST PREPARATION

*Can I prepare for Step-2 CS using only books?*
No, practice is more important than reading books. Practice is definitely the key to success.

*How many days do I need to practice before I take Step-2 CS?*
It is highly subjective since it depends on your experience and English proficiency. Practice until you get the confidence. The longer you take the more room you get for distracted and bored. If you are in touch with your clinical work, you can do it in a few weeks. Above all, you should learn time management, which is critical to pass this examination.

*How can I get a study partner while I prepare for this exam?*
chatrooms, phone, blogs

*I do not have a practice partner. What is the next best alternative to prepare for Step-2 CS?*
Form a list of questions for each case. Repeat those questions loudly to yourself. However, nobody lives in an isolated island. You will surely find a scapegoat in your spouse, friend or colleague to help you practice the cases.

*I am worrying about immunization schedule advice to parents of the young children. Can you give some advice?*
There is a nice table at *http://www.cispimmunize.org/IZSchedule_Childhood.pdf* on immunizations. Look at it a few times, you will be comfortable to answer the questions regarding immunization schedule.

*I am a bit confused about prenatal tests that should be done during the pregnancy. Can you give me some advice?*
There is a nice table at *www.hon.ch/Dossier/MotherChild/common_procedures/first_tests. html*
    Read it a few times and you will be confident

*How to overcome anxiety in Step 2 CS?*
Every one taking Step-2 CS feels anxiety before the test and frustration after the test. So, do not think you are alone on that rope. Every body taking Step-2 CS forgets to perform a few things in their encounter. So, do not run panic if you mess up the first few cases.

*How shall I make travel plans for Step 2 CS?*
If you are traveling a long distance, consider arriving at least a day before your Step 2 CS session to avoid last minute hurry. Reserve a room in the nearest motel 10 or 15 days before the exam. Check the local temperatures and pack your bag with appropriate clothing. Refer to the city guide for more information about your test center area.

*Will a drive of 9-10 hours on the day before the exam will affect my performance?*
Definitely, do not drive too long before the exam. You need to feel fresh on the day of the exam because Step-2 CS is, to some extent, a stressful test. Try to be as relaxing as possible before the examination.

# TEST CENTERS

*I live in Georgia. Can I request NBME to assign me Atlanta center?*
Yes, you can if the openings are available. Therefore, apply and register in advance to maximize your chances of taking the test at your favorite test center on your preferred date.

*Can you suggest some hotels near test center in Atlanta?*
Country Inn, Best Western, Days Inn, Econo Lodge. You can get detailed information by a simple search on Google

*I am taking my Step-2 CS in Philadelphia. Name a few motels near the test center?*
Divine Tracy Hotel, International Drive Latham Hotel, Wyndham at Franklin Plaza, Hilton Inn at Penn, Cornerstone Bed and Breakfast.

Also, Sheraton, it is 3 blocks away from the test center, they also have a discount rate for test takers. You can also go to web sites like *www.tripadvisor.com, www.orbitz. com, www.cheaphotels.com* for good deals that vary from time to time.

*I am taking my test in Chicago test center. Can you suggest some hotels near the test center for accommodation?*
Marriot hotel. Just in front of the test center

*Can I keep my luggage at the test center?*
No, you will be given only a small locker to keep your personal belongings like watch, camera, cell phone, hand bag etc. There will be no place for bigger items like suitcases.

*I don't have a personal stethoscope to take to my exam. What shall I do?*
You don't have to worry about it. The test center will provide stethescope and other devices. They will provide even a white coat. But try to take your own.

*Do I need to take my lab coat with me to the Clinical Skills test center?*
Yes, try to take your own lab coat with you to the Clinical Skills test center.

*How long do USMLE Step-2 CS administration last?*
The duration of the Step-2 CS, including orientation, testing, and breaks, is approximately eight hours.

# PATIENT ENCOUNTERS

*Can I memorize a set of questions for each case?*
No, each case is special and unique. Do not anticipate what a patient will tell you. Follow what each patient will tell you and follow from there. If you start formulating a list of questions you may fail this exam where you do not know what case you have been presented with.

*Can I wear my watch during the examination?*
No

*What time will the exam get over for a morning session?*
Around 4'o clock

*What is draping? When shall I drape the patient in Step-2 CS?*
Draping is the technique of covering the patient with a cloth in loose folds. Draping is done so that the patient might feel more comfortable during your conversation and physical examination. You sure don't want to sit right in front of them on your chair looking directly at their legs. You will see the draping cloth on the chair or stool in the examination room. Drape the patient immediately after introducing your self lest you forget to do that later. However, you will be given credit if you are able to drape the patient at any time before you start your physical examination.

*What are the things we need to do when a SP comes for pre-employment check-up?*
First do what they ask for on the paper they give you. You need not write a Patient Note for this case. So do not worry thinking about the Patient note.

　　If they ask you to measure blood pressure measure in both hands. Read carefully the instructions given in the form. You might measure blood pressure in supine position when the form asks you to do that in sitting position. Read the instructions carefully.

*How the breaks will be scheduled during Step-2 CS?*
Step-2 CS has two breaks, a 30 minute-break for lunch and a 15-minute break for coffee/snack.

*What shall I do after I read the doorway instruction sheet?*
Prepare a mental picture of the case, form a short differential diagnosis of the chief complaint and then write down—KISS RED CPR LIQORFAAA TRIFT PAMPHUGSFOSSED WPSCF—on your blank paper. Note down the chief complaint, last name of the patient

and vital signs. Read KISS RED to your self. Knock on the door and perform ISS RED in that order. Then ask CPR LIQOR FAAA TRIFT PAMP HUGS FOSSED. At first glance, this mnemonic looks lengthy and cumbersome. But if you practice it enough you will enjoy it because it will save a lot of time in the real test.

*How shall I use the scrap paper inside the examination room?*
Write down your relevant mnemonics on scrap paper after reading the doorway information. Note down all positive findings on your paper while taking history.

# HISTORY TAKING

*Shall I stand or sit while taking history?*
You can sit or stand while patient is sitting. Make sure that your patient is comfortably seated during the history taking. But never sit while the patient is standing.

*Can we write important patient findings while taking history?*
Yes, you will be provided with a pen and paper to do any writing while taking the history. Enter all positive findings in the paper. You can use this information later while writing the patient note.

*What is the most important part of Step-2 CS?*
History taking. It determines your physical examination, differential diagnosis and patient note.

*What questions shall I ask the patient who come for HIV refill?*
   1. When were you diagnosed with HIV?
   2. What medications are you taking now? Are you taking them regularly?
   3. Have you ever been diagnosed with a sexually transmitted disease?
   4. Do you have any allergies?
   5. Ask other questions from PAMPHUGSFOSSED
   6. Have you been married?
   7. How many partners do you have?
   8. What is your sexual orientation: male or female or both?
   9. Do you have any support systems to assist you?
   10. Do you drink bottled water?
   11. Did you take immunization with pneumonia vaccination?
   12. Do you have any travel plans?
   13. Have you noticed any change on your skin or mucous membranes?
   14. Do you have any ulcers on any part of your body?

*How much time shall I spend on physical examination?*
Do not spend more than five minutes on physical examination.

264

*How can we test reasoning capacity of a patient in a psychiatric case?*
Tell a proverb to the patient and ask him to interpret the meaning

*How can we test the judgmental capacity of a patient in a psychiatric case?*
Give the patient a situation to resolve.
    E.g. What would you do if you needed medical attention? or What would you do if you found an addressed envelope on the road in front of your home?

*What topics shall I inquire into when I take social history?*
Occupation & work situation
Tobacco use
Alcohol use
Recreational drug use
Home life
Environmental changes
Traveling

*Can I talk to the patient while washing my hands?*
Yes, you can turn your head toward the patient and ask any questions, for example, "Mr. Roberts, do you have any concerns to share with me?"
    Or "Mr. Christopher, I forgot to ask you, have you ever been told that you have a heart murmur?"
    You can be as lively as possible. But your conversation should not make you forget to dry your hands after washing. Never touch the patient with wet hands.

# PHYSICAL EXAMINATION

*How do I use the leg rest and foot-step of the patient examination table . . . are they simple?*
Very simple, they'll show you how to use the examination table before commencing the test. You have ample time to practice with a sample examination table. Adjust the foot-rest when you need to have the patient get down from the table to check their gait.

*I never used an ophthalmoscope before in my medical training. I am worrying how I could manage it in the examination?*
They will demonstrate the ophthalmoscope before the session starts. Practice how to use the ophthalmoscope for a few minutes. Sticking it in front of the SP's eye in a standard manner is enough to get the point rather than worrying about whether or not you can visualize the retina.

*Do I need to do a general or a focussed physical examination?*
In Step 2 CS, trying to do a general physical examination is a straight road to the pit of failure. Just perform a focussed physical examination. You will have only 15 minutes

to spend with the patient. Therefore, try to finish history in 8 minutes, focused physical examination in 5 minutes and counseling in 2 minutes.

*If a patient reports tenderness on superficial palpation, do we need to do deep palpation or rebound tenderness at the same site?*
Yes, positive findings on superficial palpation do not exclude the necessity of deep palpation. However, you need to reassure the patient that you will be gentle, apologize for hurting and explain the importance of the deep palpation before continuing with deep palpation and other tests. Because you are dealing with a Standardized Patient you are not really hurting any one, speaking as it is!

*How can I do a mental status examination in a patient with signs of depression?*
Do only Mini-Mental Status Examination. There is no time for extensive examination

*How much time shall I spend on auscultation of the heart and lungs?*
Spend 2 to 3 seconds on each spot and while listening think what you want to do next.

*Do patients exhibit abnormal physical findings in Step-2 CS?*
Yes, patients will be instructed to act out certain abnormal physical findings while you are doing the physical examination. E.g. patient with acute appendicitis will shout with pain while you are pressing in the right lower quadrant. Patient with acute cholecystitis complain that it is painful when you are pressing in his right upper quadrant. Patients with lung consolidation will be instructed to say 99 loudly when you are approaching the lower lobes while performing the bronchophony.

*How do we test for nystagmus?*
Ask the patient to look at your finger and move your finger around the sideways in the form of H

*Should we check for sensation in face while doing CNS-5th nerve examination?*
Yes, but do not spend much time on this.

*Do I need to measure the size of the liver using a scale in case of hepatomegaly. Or is it enough to just percuss the upper and lower borders and make a rough estimate of liver size? Do they provide us with a ruler/scale for measurement?*
You just need to percuss, you do not need to measure. You will not be provided any scale and you *should not* make any pen marks on the patient's body.

*Should we do Rinnie and Weber tests in all CNS cases?*
No, do those tests only if the patient presents with a complaint of hearing loss

*Do we need to examine CNS in a patient with hiccups?*
Yes, a brain stem tumor could present with hiccups.

*How can I pursue a female patient before auscultating the heart and lungs?*
Say, *"Mrs. Harvey, could you please lift your left breast so that I can listen your heart sounds"*—then auscultate over the PMI. You are allowed to keep the diaphragm of your stethoscope between the two breasts during auscultation. However, you are not allowed to palpate any areas that involve breast tissue.

*What clinical instruments are available in the examination room?*
Ophthalmoscope
Otoscope
Tuning forks
Reflex hammer
BP apparatus
Nasal speculum
Tongue depressor
Gloves
Sticks
Cotton buds

*Are we allowed to examine axillary lymph nodes?*
Yes, you can palpate axillary or inguinal lymph nodes if you think it is necessary.

*Do I have to do PERRLA in all patients?*
Yes, but don't spend more than 6-7 seconds on it

*What systems do we need to examine in a patient with depression?*
Thyroid, MMSE, heart and lungs

*In Step-2 CS, will we have to be doing any rectal or breast exams?*
No, you are not allowed to do

1. Corneal reflex examination
2. Breast examination
3. Pelvic examination
4. Anal examination

To compensate that you can tell to the patient that those examinations are required for your diagnosis in physical examination as part of your diagnostic work up.

*I know there is not enough time to do everything in Step 2 CS. But, do you recommend measuring blood pressure at least in both upper limbs of every patient?*
Measuring blood pressure, recording temperatures on thermometer, measuring the height and weight of the patient are suicidal attempts in this test. You will hardly have time for these things. Almost for all patients, you will be provided with their blood pressure, temperature, pulse and respiratory rate measurements and in some cases, more information. In some cases like pre-employment check-up you will be specifically asked to measure the blood pressure. Unless you are specifically asked to measure the blood pressure, simply take the given values on the door way information sheet as accurate measurements.

*I don't know how to do Tilt table test. Do I have to learn it?*
No need. You won't be able to do this test in Step 2 CS

*How to vibrate a tuning fork?*
Hold the tuning fork at the tip and hit your palm with it quickly.

*What shall I do when I run out of time while doing the physical examination?*
If you are running out of time, try to give a good closure to the encounter instead of doing a few more physical examination maneuvers. A good closure to the patient encounter is very essential.

*While estimating liver span, do we have to mark it on patient's abdomen?*
No, never mark on the patient in Clinical Skills examination.

*What systems do we need to examine in a diabetic patient?*
Sensory system—pinprick, vibration
Reflexes
Fundoscopy
Peripheral pulses in all extremities

*If a patient has a painful shoulder how shall I start my physical examination?*
First examine the normal shoulder then go for the painful shoulder. This rule applies to all joints as well.

*Do I need to do a full cardiac examination in all cases?*
No. If it is connected directly with cardiac system, do a complete cardiac exam both in sitting and supine position. For other diseases, just listen to the heart at 3 or 4 areas, 3 seconds per area.

*Do I need to wear gloves for physical examination?*
No need, wearing gloves kills time and you won't be able to take notes on your blank paper, if you want to, comfortably. So proceed with bare hands.

# COUNSELING & CLOSURE

*Should we discuss the treatment and prognosis with the patient?*
Most Step-2 CS cases will end up with more than one possible disease. You are not sure what the diagnosis is at that point. Therefore, do not discuss the treatment and prognosis to the patient at this stage. But, never mention your treatment plans or referrals in your patient note.

*What shall I tell the patient if I do not know the answer to his question?*
*"Mr. Questioner, I appreciate you asked me that question. But I do not know the answer at this point. I might be able to refer other sources and give you an exact answer as soon as possible. All right?"*

*How can I tell a patient that he/she might have dementia?*
Mr. Patient, I think you may have a decrease in the function of your brain, most probably due to Alzheimer disease or multiinfarct dementia. These diseases might cause mainly memory problems and other impairments in your physical activities.

*Will I be required to diagnose and treat real patients?*
No. The Step-2 CS consists of encounters with standardized patients(SPs), lay persons trained to accurately and consistently portray patients. The SPs will respond to your questions with answers appropriate to the case and, upon physical examination, will demonstrate appropriate physical findings. You will be expected to proceed through each encounter with an SP as you would with a real patient, but you should not do treatment of any kind.

# PATIENT NOTE

*How shall I use scrap paper for writing the patient note?*
While taking history from the patient, write the pertinent findings on your scrap or blank paper. This information will be useful to write your patient note. Scrap paper is your main guide for writing the patient note. Record the patient's name, chief complaint, vital signs and all positive findings on the scrap paper. Record all positive findings from the scrap paper on your patient note.

*Should I write my Patient Note on paper or type into the computer?*
It depends on your skills. If you have good typing speed or bad hand writing, go for computer

# TEST RESULTS

*Should I apply for a recheck of my result in Step-2 CS?*
I think you are wasting your money.

*I failed my Step 2 CS. What should I do?*

Don't give up. Many students who failed Step 2 CS passed it later and now joined residency programs. You should identify the mistakes you committed, rectify them and practice the cases in timed mode.

Note: If you have any unanswered questions, please contact www.usmle.org or www.ecfmg. org. Also, refer www.nbme.org for the latest information about USMLE Step-2 CS.

Printed in the United Kingdom by
Lightning Source UK Ltd., Milton Keynes
138015UK00001B/88/P